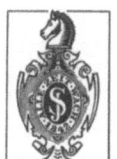

M. J. Halhuber · R. Günther · M. Ciresa

ECG
An Introductory Course

A Practical Introduction
to Clinical Electrocardiography

With the Assistance of
P. Schumacher and W. Newesely

English Translation of the Sixth German Edition
by H. J. Hirsch

With 98 Figures

Springer-Verlag
Berlin Heidelberg New York 1979

Prof. Dr. med. M. J. HALHUBER, Klinik Höhenried für Herz-
und Kreislaufkrankheiten, D-8131 Bernried/Starnberger See

Prof. Dr med. R. GÜNTHER, Medizinische Universitätsklinik,
A-6020 Innsbruck

Prim. Dr. med. M. CIRESA, Bezirkskrankenhaus, A-6130 Schwaz

Dr. med P. SCHUMACHER, Pediatrician, A-6020 Innsbruck

Ing. W. NEWESELY, Technical Consultant, A-6020 Innsbruck

Translator: H. J. HIRSCH, M. B., B. Ch., F. R. C. Path., London

Title of the original edition: EKG-Einführungskurs.
Eine praktische Propädeutik der klinischen Elektrokardiographie. 6th edition.
Springer-Verlag Berlin Heidelberg New York 1978

The 1st to 4th German edition were published under the title "Praktischer EKG-Kurs"
by J. A. Barth, Munich

ISBN-13: 978-3-540-09326-8   e-ISBN-13: 978-3-642-67280-4
DOI: 10.1007/978-3-642-67280-4

Library of Congress Cataloging in Publication Data. Halhuber, Max J., ECG, an
introductory course. Translation of EKG-Einführungskurs. Bibliography: p.   Includes
index. 1. Electrocardiography. I. Günther, R., 1922- joint author. II. Ciresa, M., 1929-
joint author.
III. Title RC683.5.E5H2813 616.1'2'0754 79-9900

Typesetting, printing, and binding: Oscar Brandstetter Druckerei KG, 6200 Wiesbaden.
2120/3130-543210

Preface

Since 1955, we have conducted an annual one-week ECG course at Innsbruck. This book represents a summary of our didactic experience.

This English translation follows the enlarged sixth German edition. It contains many diagrams and new examples of tracings, such as the orthogonal leads system of Frank, explanation of extreme axis deviation by the hemiblock concept, atrioventricular conduction disorders (His bundle electrogram), re-entry mechanisms, and the exercise ECG.

The limits and dangers of ECG interpretations that, in our opinion, should be emphasized in an introductory presentation, are summarized in a final chapter.

Our main aim was to make indigestible material palatable to the beginner; to provide him with a red thread through the labyrinth of ECG patterns by adopting a uniform approach, namely vectorial interpretation, in order to understand especially difficult areas (e. g. the differential diagnosis of infarction) by means of simplified diagrams; and to prepare him for the study of systematic textbooks. We believe that many such books should be read in order to comprehend a subject that is generally considered difficult by physicians and at the same time to promote critical understanding when called upon to evaluate an ECG in practice.

The following publications to which we ourselves owe valuable suggestions, even if they are not explicitly mentioned in our text, are recommended:

BELZ, G. G., STAUCH, M.: Notfall-EKG-Fibel, 2nd ed. Berlin, Heidelberg, New York: Springer 1977

BÜCHNER, C. H., DRÄGERT, W.: Schrittmachertherapie des Herzens. Mannheim: Boehringer 1973

CABRERA, E.: Electrocardiographie clinique. Paris: Masson 1959

FRIEDMANN, H. H.: Outline of electrocardiography. New York, Toronto, London: McGraw-Hill 1963

GOLDMAN, M. J.: Principles of clinical electrocardiography, 9th ed. Los Altos: Lange Medical Publ. 1976

HEINECKER, R.: EKG in Praxis und Klinik, 10th ed. Stuttgart: Thieme 1975

HEINECKER, R.: EKG-Quiz, 2nd ed. Stuttgart: Thieme 1974

HOLZMANN, M.: Klinische Elektrokardiographie, 5th ed. Stuttgart: Thieme 1965

LEMMERZ, A. H.: Das orthogonale EKG-Ableitungssystem nach Frank im Routinebetrieb, 4th ed. Basel, Munich, Paris, London, New York, Sydney: Karger 1973

LEMMERZ, A. H.: Atlas des EKG nach Frank. Basel, Munich, Paris, London New York, Sydney: Karger 1970

LEMMERZ, A. H., SCHMIDT, R.: Registrierfehler in der EKG-Praxis. Stuttgart: Thieme 1964

LENEGRE, J., CAROUSO, O., CHEVALIER, H.: Electrocardiographie clinique. Paris: Masson 1954

LUTTEROTTI V., M., KORTH, C.: Atlas der klinischen Elektrokardiographie, 3rd ed. Munich, Berlin: Urban & Schwarzenberg 1963

NETTER, F. H.: The Ciba collection of medical illustrations, Vol. V: Heart. New York: Ciba 1969

RITTER, O., FATTORUSSO, V.: Atlas der Elektrokardiographie, 4th ed. Basel: Karger 1974

SCHAUB, F. A.: Grundriss der klinischen Elektrokardiographie. Basel: Geigy 1965

SCHLANDT, R. C., HURST, J. W.: Advances in electrocardiography. New York, London: Grune & Stratton 1972

SCHWEIZER, W.: Einführung in die Kardiologie. Bern, Stuttgart, Vienna: Huber 1972

SO, C. S.: Praktische Elektrokardiographie. Munich: Selecta 1974

SODI-PALLARES, D.: Le nuove basi della elettrocardiografia. Padova: Piccin 1959

WIRTZFELD, A., BAEDEKER, W. B.: Rhythmusstörungen des Herzens. Munich, Berlin, Vienna: Urban & Schwarzenberg 1974

The following literature is recommended for further reading.

ARMSTRONG, M. L.: Electrocardiograms. A systematic method of reading, 4th ed. Chicago: Year Book Medical Publ. 1978

BECKWITH, J.: Grant's Clinical Electrocardiography. New York: McCraw Hill 1970

CHUNG, E. K.: Ambulatory Electrocardiography. Berlin, Heidelberg, New York: Springer 1979

CHUNG, E. K.: ECG Diagnosis. New York: Harper & Row 1977

FRIEDEN/RUBIN: ECG Case Studies. Bern, Stuttgart, Wien: Huber

FRIEDMAN, H.: Diagnostic Electrocardiography and Vectorcardiography, 2nd ed. New York: McCraw Hill 1977

GOLDBERGER, A.: Clinical Electrocardiography. St. Louis: Mosby 1977

HURST, J. W., MYERBURG, R. J.: Introduction to Electrography. New York: McGraw Hill 1973

LYON, L.: Basic Electrocardiography Handbook. New York: Van Nostrand Reinhold 1977

MANGIOLA, St.: Self-Assessment in Electrocardiography. Philadelphia: Lippincott 1977

diography. New York: Oxford University Press 1976

PIPBERGER, H. V.: Computer Analysis of the Electrocardiogram (Einthoven-Lecture). Leiden: University Press 1975

REDDY, C. V., GOULD, L. A.: Correlative Atlas of Vectorcardiograms and ECG. New York: Futura Publ. 1977

SCHAMROTH, L.: An Introduction to Electrocardiography. Philadelphia: Lippincott 1971

STEIN, E.: The Electrocardiogram. Philadelphia: Saunders 1976

Quotations, individual articles, special publications and names of authors in text and figures have been dispensed with, since their inclusion would encroach on the clarity of the information to be acquired and also disproportionately exceed the dimension of an introductory course.

The Authors

Sources of the Figures

Fig. 23–25: Modified according to W. Schweizer: Einführung in die Kardiologie, 2. Aufl. Bern, Stuttgart, Wien: Huber 1979

Fig. 37, 41: Modified according to Ritter/Fattorusso: Atlas der Elektrokardiographie, 5. Aufl. Basel: Karger 1976

Fig. 38, 39, 42, 57: According to Friedman, H. H., Outline of Electricardiography, New York, Toronto, London: McGraw Hill 1963

Fig. 40, 43, 46, 47, 48, 49: Modified according to A. Wirtzfeld und W. D. Baldeker; Rhythmusstörungen des Herzens. München, Berlin, Wien: Urban & Schwarzenberg 1974

Fig. 14: According to M. J. Goldman: Principles of Clinical Electrocardiography. Los Altos: Lange Medical Publ. 1976

Fig. 81, 82, 83, 84, 87, 88, 95, 96: Burch, G. E., Winsor, T.; A primer of Electrocardiography. Philadelphia: Lea & Febiger 1971

Contents

1. Vectorcardiography

For didactic reasons, a uniform approach to the electrophysiologic action of the heart will be maintained in all sections of this book, namely the vector hypothesis, whose basis is the dipole theory. Thus, other theoretical explanations of the ECG action currents, e. g., difference construction, are not necessarily rejected as incorrect. It is only a didactic simplification that makes introduction to clinical electrocardiography easier for the beginner, as experience shows.

In this introductory chapter, a few principles of electrophysiology will be discussed as far as is necessary for understanding clinical electrocardiography and correct interpretation of tracings.

The electrophysiology of the heart can easily be demonstrated by the electric properties of a single heart muscle fiber at rest, during spread (depolarization), and during regression (repolarization) of a stimulus. The concept of dipole and vector will be discussed thereafter.

Many energy conversions are known to be associated with changes in the electric state. Thus, excitation of a muscle fiber provokes electric phenomena even before mechanical contraction sets in. In the heart, an electric stimulus precedes the mechanical systole by a fraction of a second. Since stimulation of the vast myofibrillar syncytium of the heart spreads in different directions and is very complex, a single muscle fiber will be used as a model for simple explanation of all electric actions and the study of stimulus conduction. The important so-called third bioelectric principle should be remembered:

A stimulated muscle area is electrically negative compared with an unstimulated area.' A muscle fiber at rest is called *polarized*.

Bioelectr. principle

If a fiber is stimulated, say at its left end (Fig. 1), whether mechanically, chemically, or electrically, the wave of excitation spreads over the fiber in a fraction of a second. The permeability of the membrane is suddenly and transiently much increased at the site of the stimulus, which develops the negative charge of the interior of the fiber for a brief period.

The process of enhanced permeability of the cell membrane during excitation is called *depolarization*. A potential gradient arises on the outside between negative charge of the stimulated and positive charge of the as yet not stimulated area of the fiber (Fig. 1). These differences in potential are the cause of a current, the so-called action current. It flows from the still unstimulated fiber surface to stimulated portions. If two electrodes are placed on the fiber surface (Fig. 2), this "axial current" can be measured with a galvanometer. As long as the fiber remains unstimulated, no difference of potential exists between points a and b,

Depolarization

Action current

1

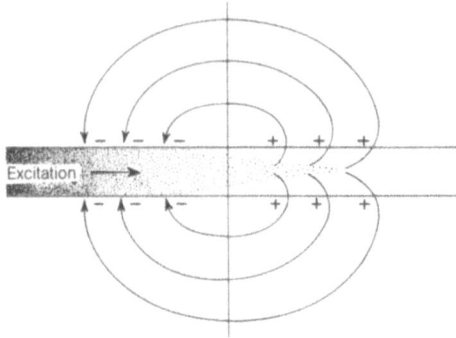

Fig. 1. Spread of excitation in a muscle fiber

and the galvanometer shows no deflection. But as soon as activation from point a flows through the fiber, point a is electronegative relative to point b. The swing of the galvanometer reflects the degree of potential difference (voltage), and the electrogram on the right represents the change of the potential difference in time between points a and b diagrammatically. As soon as the action current has covered the whole muscle fiber and this is depolarized evenly, there is no longer any

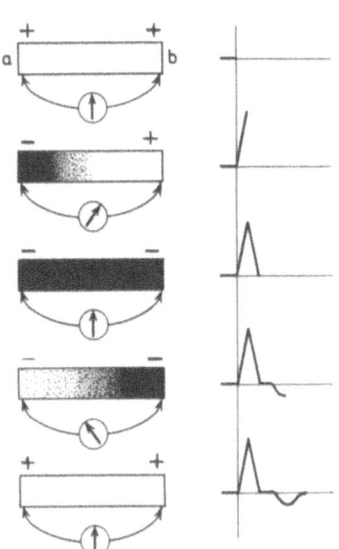

Fig. 2. Depolarization and repolarization of a muscle fiber

potential difference between points a and b, the action current has ceased, and deflection returns to the base line. Therefore, if the whole fiber is stimulated, only a negative charge exists at the outside, and no potential difference is measurable — as at rest. Only on regressing excitation — *repolarization* — does a gradient of potential recur. If repolarization starts again from point a, that is the left extremity of the fiber where depolarization also began, the gradient of potential is opposite to that of depolarization. For this time, point a is electropositive against point b. Since regression of activation, repolarization, takes a different path and is slower than depolarization, the final deflection (T) differs from the main wave (R). As soon as repolarization, i. e., regression of the stimulus of the muscle fiber, is completed, a potential difference between points a and b no longer exists and galvanometer and tracing revert to their position at rest or on the zero line.

If we imagine our model of a muscle fiber to be in saline in a Petri dish, the stimulated muscle fiber activates this medium like an electric field, causing a potential difference between two neighboring points. Physicists call this approximation of two opposed charges a dipole. When the wave of excitation in a muscle fiber spreads, the negative charge of the stimulated area pushes the positive charge of the as yet unstimulated area in front of it, as it were. At their meeting point, the two charges form a dipole (see also Fig. 4, where excitation of a single muscle fiber is transferred to the heart in Einthoven's triangle).

The distribution of the potential produced by the dipole "muscle fiber" is called the electric field of the dipole. All points of identical potential lie on so-called isopotential lines (Figs. 3 and 4). If the process of stimulation of a single muscle fiber is compared with the heart as the sum of many fiber excitations and one equates the conducting milieu with surrounding tissues in the body, the various potential differences during spread of the excitation in the heart can be derived with electrodes from the body surface just as from the edge of the saline solution in the Petri dish.

The effects of this dipole or the muscle fiber on the electric field depend on position, direction, and magnitude of the charge of the dipole. There is no difference in potential between any points on a straight line that passes perpendicularly through the center of the dipole along the dipole axis. This line with the potential 0 (zero) divides the electric field — assumed to be circular — into a positive half, containing the positive "head" of the dipole, and a negative half, where the "tail" of the dipole is situated. The closer an electrode is approached to the positive or negative dipole termination at the edge of the field, the greater becomes the positive or negative deflection of the galvanometer or electrocardiograph. The greatest potentials are those in the longitudinal direction of the dipole or its electric axis; the smallest are found near the base line that is perpendicular to the electric axis. Figure 3 shows why in the above example, the galvanometer indicates the potential

3

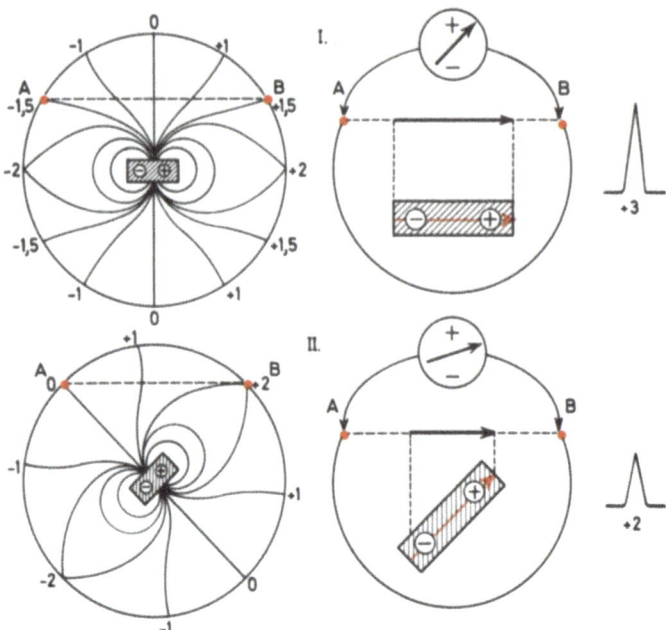

Fig. 3. Dipole in an electric field

differences between points A and B from 3 (it joins two points that lie on the isopotential lines −1.5 and +1.5). In the lower example, the galvanometer registers a minor deflection 2, since it connects point A, that lies on the isopotential line 0, and perpendicular to the electric axis of the dipole, with point B of the isopotential line +2, that lies on the electric axis. In Fig. 4, our model of the muscle fiber or the dipole has been transferred to the human heart. Obviously, this imaginary aid is only partly applicable:

1. The excitation processes in the heart cannot readily be compared with an individual muscle fiber. But, considered from a corresponding electrode interspace, its electric property resembles several single light sources that are perceived as *one* light from the distance.

2. The body is not an ideal homogeneous medium; its tissues have different conducting powers. But experience teaches that this difference in conduction is practically negligible.

3. The dipole "heart" does not lie ideally in the center of a spherical homogeneous conductor; however, the distance heart-limb remains fairly constant and is roughly equidistant from the proximal portions of the upper and lower extremities. Hence, the so-called triangle of Einthoven could be constructed from the lines of conduction. Instead of

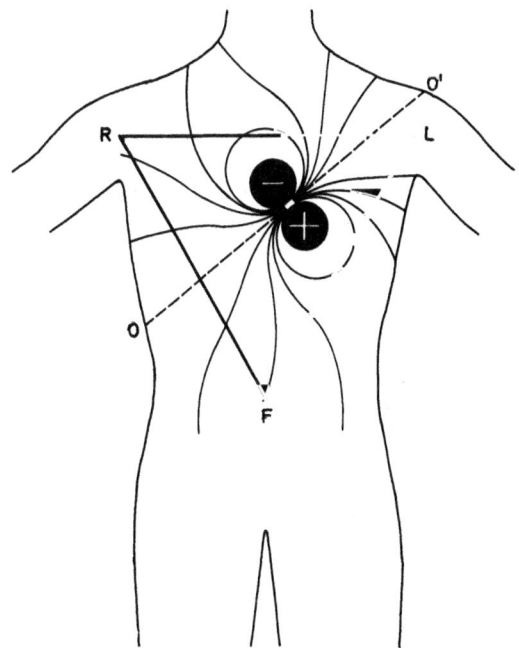

Fig. 4. The heart as dipole in an electric field (body) with Einthoven's triangle

the conduction line A-B, where the electrodes for measuring the potential difference were placed in Fig. 3, the lead between R = right arm and L = left arm may be employed, that is lead I of the bipolar leads, by which the potential differences between points R and L is measured.

The isopotential lines of the dipole "heart" have been drawn into the electric field "body" in Fig. 4. Since it would be impractical to construct the different lines of potential in the electric field, the vector concept greatly simplifies matters.

An entity that is determined by only one quantity is a *scalar* one (weight, temperature, etc), whereas one that requires for its definition quantity and direction, is a *vectorial* entity. For instance, electromotor power is a vectorial entity; it arises from quantity and direction, and can be represented by a *vector*. Vector concept

A vector is a segment of a line with the following properties: Vector character-
a) It has a starting and an end point. istics
b) It occupies a position, namely that of the line that carries it, also called "vector carrier". If the line has direction, it is called axis.
c) It has a sense of direction, like an imaginary shot from starting to end point.

5

d) It has a length or a quantity, that is the distance between starting and end point of the vector, measured by a predetermined unit. This unit, designated + or −, is the numerical component of the vector in relation to its axis.

The directional magnitude is represented by an arrow, which indicates the direction of the spread of excitation in the muscle fiber (dipole) with the conducting medium (body). Its position is determined by the position of the charges that it connects, and its magnitude (in units of length) corresponds with the magnitude of the difference potential between the poles (in units of difference potential = mV). It is internationally agreed that the head of the vector always points to the positive pole. Since the main direction of a stimulus in the heart runs from the base to the apex, the largest vector adopts this direction during cardiac stimulation. Projected onto the frontal plane, it corresponds approximately to the anatomic heart axis. It is not a sole vector, but, with the mass of muscle fibers that form the heart, it represents the summation or integral vector, the sum of all the main directions of excitation of numerous small individual vectors. But even this is not precise enough, for the time factor has been neglected. Hence we have to add: it is an integral or summation vector at a certain moment of cardiac stimulation. Obviously, this dipole or vector has a different magnitude and direction at any moment of stimulus conduction in the heart; today, it is directly registered by vectorcardiography. Whereas the ECG reflects a

Vector-
cardiogram

changing potential — always between two points — in time, the vectorcardiogram records a loop comprising all vector tips during a cardiac cycle (Fig. 5).

Vector

The task of vectorcardiography is to find a system of three leads (three axes) that permit construction of the components of the cardiac

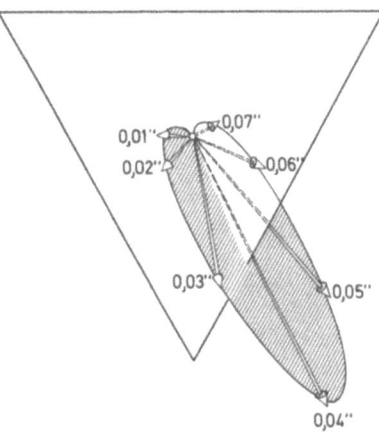

Fig. 5. Vector loop

vector in three dimensions. The magnitude of the resulting cardiac vector and its direction in space will thus determine each phase of cardiac action.

Does representation of spatial processes of vectorcardiography, that is the projection of the spatial peripheral loop around all vectors in three planes, offer an advantage over the information provided by vectorial interpretation of the ECG? In principle, this is impossible, since the components of the vectorcardiogram always are two ECGs. But the discussion on the advantages of vectorcardiography over ECG has not been concluded. It was shown that in certain cases ECG diagnosis is favorably complemented and detailed by vectorcardiography. Causes advanced are: greater descriptiveness of the vectorcardiogram, particularly as regards demonstration of spatial bioelectric processes; second, the fact that these processes are presented in the ECG in such a manner that they do less justice to actual conditions than vectorcardiography — due to the leads employed in conventional electrocardiography; and finally, the fact that the ECG is uncharacteristic because of opposed bioelectric mechanisms in some cases, where the vectorcardiogram still permits typical changes to be recognized for both mechanisms (e. g., left and right ventricular hypertrophy, bundle branch block, and myocardial infarct).

2. Usual ECG Leads and Their Interrelation

Just as electrodes can be applied to the border of an electric medium in whose center an excited muscle fiber is present, and different potentials are measured with a galvanometer (Fig. 3), those potentials produced by the heart muscle can be obtained from the surface of the human body. Ever since Einthoven, the points of application have been the arms and the left lower limb (the right is also used) (Fig. 4). Arms and legs act only as conducting cables, hence the electrodes can be applied to forearm or leg without drawbacks.

Standard or bipolar leads of Einthoven
The triangle of Einthoven is formed by the three electrode points on the right arm, left arm, and left leg. It is an equilateral triangle whose sides are known as leads. Lead I lies between the electrodes of right and left arm, lead II between right arm and left leg, and lead III between left arm and left leg. The projection of a vector onto the individual leads in the heart is attained by dropping a perpendicular. Conversely, the respective vector may be constructed from the peak of a wave of action currents in two leads (Fig. 6). Projection of a vector is greatest if the latter is parallel with the lead, whereas it becomes smaller with increasing angle between vector and lead. If the lead is perpendicular to the vector, it is seen as a point.

The Einthoven leads lie in the frontal plane of the body. They are called *bi*polar, since they measure the difference potential between two electrodes (Fig. 7 a).

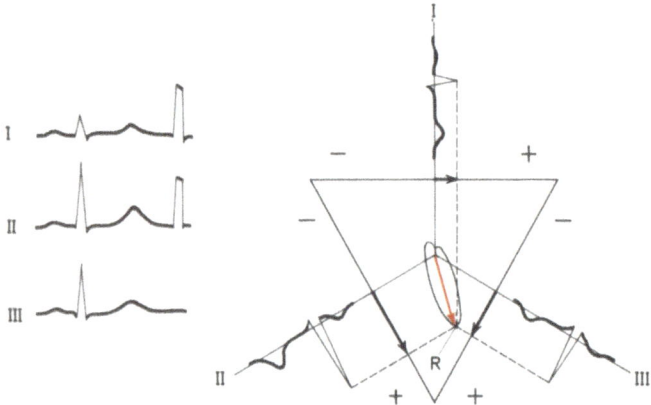

Fig. 6. R vector projection

8

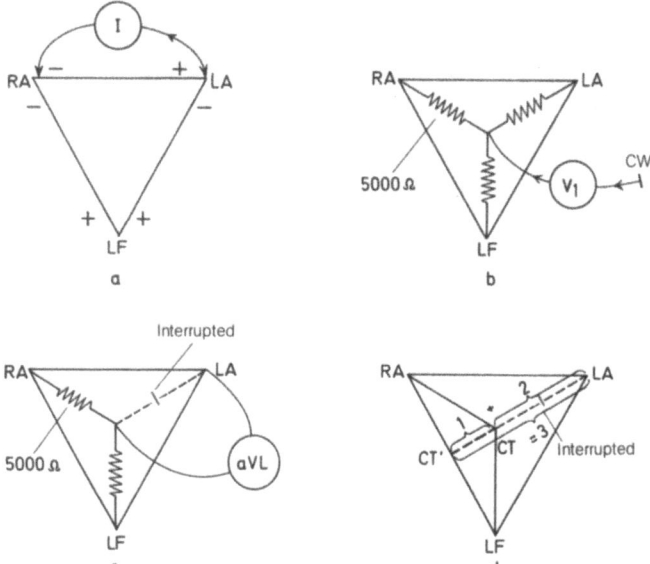

Fig. 7a–d. Evolution of unipolar leads

By interpolating high-ohmic resistors between the limb leads, Wilson obtained an electrode that lies in the center of Einthoven's triangle (Fig. 7b), which he called "central terminal". This indifferent electrode can also be imagined to lie at the zero point of the dipole between positive and negative charge. Rotation of the dipole around this zero point does not affect the position of the 0 electrode. Since it was shown that the ECG waves, which are written with an exploring electrode against this 0 electrode, are smaller than those of the standard leads, which derive their voltage from two different electrodes (Fig. 7a), they were augmented by Goldberger, who interrupted the lead connecting the exploring electrode and the 0 electrode (Fig. 7c). For instance, if aVL is to be written, the 0 point (CT) is displaced to the center of the lead between right arm and left leg (CT′) due to this interruption. Figure 7d shows that this shift of the 0 point from CT to CT′ creates an augmentation of lead VL (voltage left arm) — originally lying between CT (central terminal) and LA (left arm) — in a ratio of 3 : 2 and 1 · 5 : 1. The consequence is the augmented lead aVL of Goldberger. The waves of this derivation are about as large as those obtained by bipolar standard leads.

Figure 8a–c shows points of application of the standard leads according to Einthoven (a), the unipolar leads of Goldberger (b), and the unipolar precordial leads of Wilson (c).

"Central terminal" of Wilson

9

Goldberger's leads could also be called "bipolar" leads from which potential differences are measured between two electrodes one of which has an almost 0 potential. Thus, the Goldberger leads are directed toward the zero point (0 potential) in the center of the Einthoven triangle, and form an angle of 30° with its sides (standard leads).

In this manner, six leads are obtained in the frontal plane which are shifted against each other always by 30°, except a VR, which lies at the level of the right arm. This permits observation of the electric processes in the heart from various angles.

By simplifying the construction, all six leads of the frontal plane can be made to arise from the center of the heart or Wilson's central terminal (zero point of the dipole). For this purpose, the standard leads (sides of the triangle of Einthoven) are displaced parallel through the heart center (Fig. 9 a). If a circle is drawn around the triangle, the points of leads I, II, and III must be entered where the leads — parallel-displaced through the center — intersect the circumference of the circle. The standard leads have been converted to "unipolar" leads by this geometric construction, since they thus also originate at the zero point in the heart center. No essential error has been committed, since the overall orientation in the frontal plane remains unchanged. Now, all vector projections of this
triaxial system can be marked in the frontal plane; this particularly facilitates determination of the position of the heart. Transferred to the body, lead aVL lies at the left shoulder, lead I left horizontal, II at the

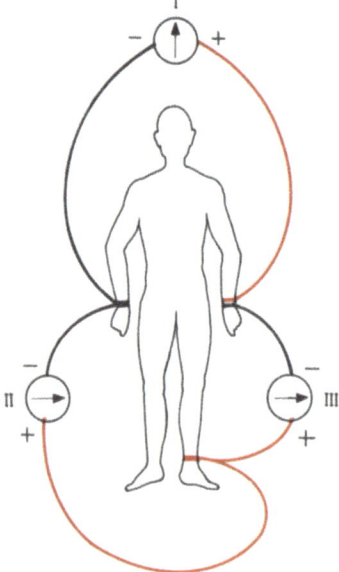

Fig. 8a

10

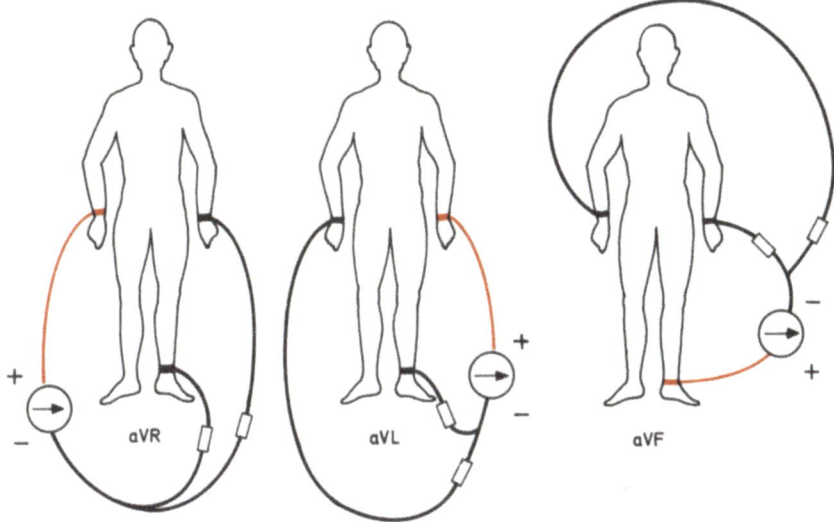

Fig. 8b

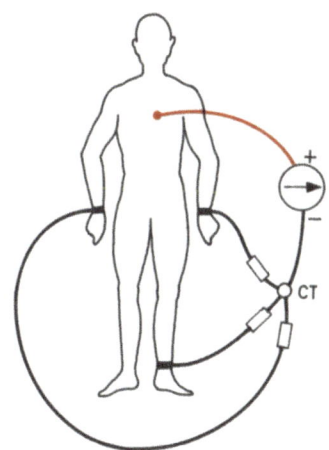

Fig. 8c

upper leg, aVF at the mons pubis in midline, III at the upper right leg, and aVR at the right shoulder. If the upper portion of the circle is divided anticlockwise in $-180°$, beginning with lead I (± 0 degree), then aVL lies at $-30°$ and aVR at $-150°$. Similarly, the lower half of the circle is divided in $+180°$, but clockwise. Lead II comes to lie at $+60°$, lead aVF at $+90°$, and lead III at $+120°$ (Fig. 9b and c).

11

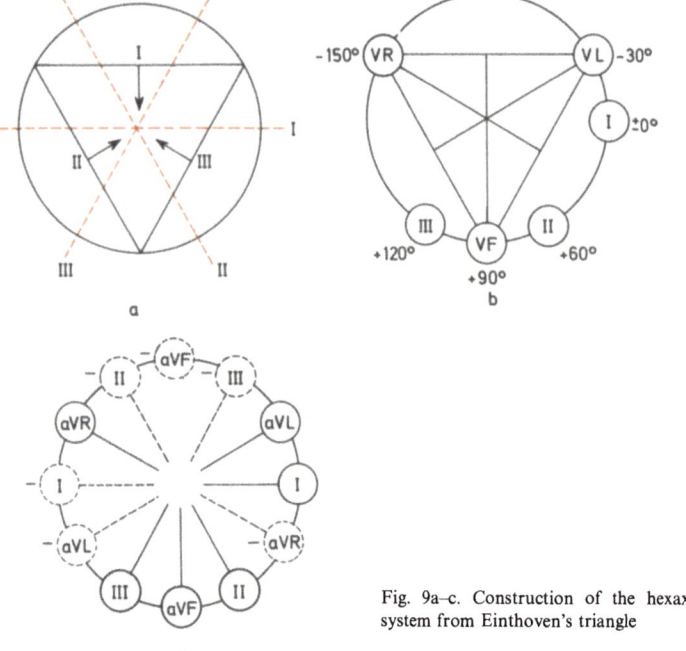

Fig. 9a–c. Construction of the hexaxial system from Einthoven's triangle

Order of extremity leads

This commonly applied sequence and polarization of limb leads is historically founded, but could be improved by a simple change of the wiring system of the ECG equipment, in order to close the gap between 0° and +60° by an electrode at +30° (−aVR).

Considering polarization and topography of leads, the extremity ones thus occupy a regular sequence (Fig. 10).

In Italy, equipment was first wired to permit writing the ECG program in the order mentioned. German manufacturers will supplement their sets if desired.

It remains to be hoped that these occasional attempts will bear fruit, and it appears certain that evaluation is facilitated not only for the beginner but also that many a so-called electrocardiographic phenomenon will be resolved.

Chest leads or Wilson leads

In order better to understand and determine the spatial vectors in the heart, projection on the horizontal plane and application of electrodes in a horizontal plane are necessary, apart from projection on the frontal plane. This enables one to detect also those vectors that lie perpendicular to the frontal plane but are not projected to it.

Figure 11 shows the position of the electrodes at the margin of the horizontal plane, designated by V1-6 (V for voltage). The electrodes are put on the chest. Again, these are unipolar leads that are written with the exploring electrode according to the diagram of Fig. 7b. Since they lie close to the heart, their deflections are greater than those of the limb

12

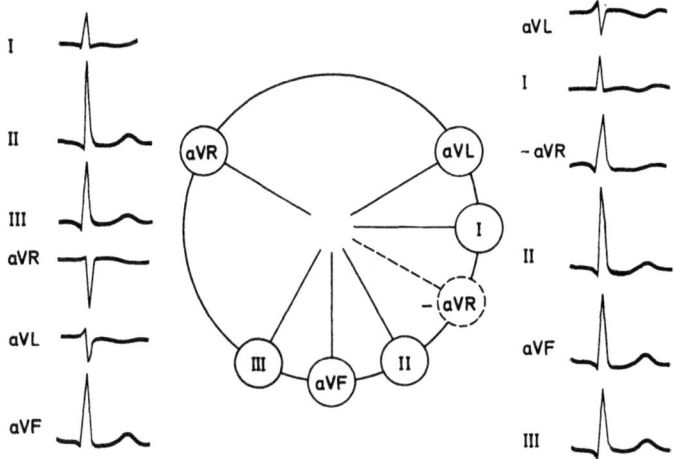

Fig. 10. Proposal for an improved order of limb lead registration

leads; hence, they need not be augmented. Figure 12 shows that V1 is applied in the right 4th ICS (intercostal space) parasternally, V2 similarly left parasternally, V3 between V2 and V4, V4 in the midclavicular line level with the apex beat (if not palpable, level with the 5th ICS), V5 at the same level as V4 in the anterior axillary line, and finally V6 at the same level in midaxillary line. Obviously, many electrodes can be applied to the right and left thorax, but 6 leads usually suffice. If the leads are extended to the right, V3 corresponds to V3r on the right chest wall (V1r = V2, V2r = V1). *Position of chest electrodes*

The triangle of Nehb tries to record from the heart in an oblique plane by leads derived from the Einthoven triangle (Fig. 13). If the Einthoven triangle is elevated anteriorly at its lower corner (application on left leg), it tilts around the assumedly fixed corner at the right shoulder into the thorax with its corner at the left shoulder and engulfs the heart. The point of electrode application at the left leg (green) will then lie over the apex, that of the left arm (yellow) at the same level in the posterior axillary line, and only that of the right arm (red) is slightly displaced, namely at the sternal insertion of the 2nd right rib. Thus, Nehb lead A (anterior) corresponds with limb lead II, Nehb lead I (inferior) with limb lead III, and Nehb lead D (dorsal) with limb lead I. *Nehb's triangle (bipolar chest leads)*

Nehb's leads A and I are suitable additional diagnostic aids in anterior and lateral wall infarction. However, most important is lead D for diagnosis of posterior wall infarct.

Esophageal leads are written with the precordial electrode It is introduced into the esophagus like a probe at different distances from *Esophageal leads*

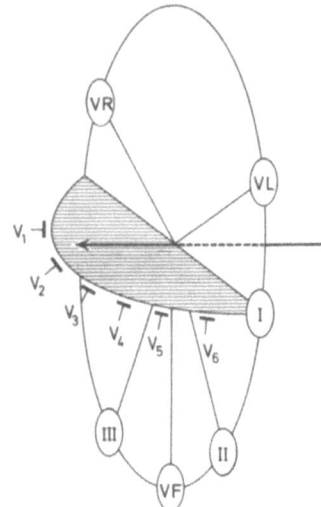

Fig. 11. Leads in the horizontal plane

the upper row of teeth (Fig. 14). It first overlies the left atrium, and the lower it is dropped, the more it lies on the posterior and inferior wall of the heart. Once the probe is in the stomach, the vectorial action of the posterior and diaphragmatic wall of the heart (e. g. posterior wall infarct) is well registered. They are also of interest for action currents in atrium, since they are closely apposed to the atrium. The tracing thus obtained is the EAG (electroatriogram). It resembles the ECG of the ventricle, which could be described as EVG (electroventriculogram). The EAG is specially distinct in complete atrioventricular block.

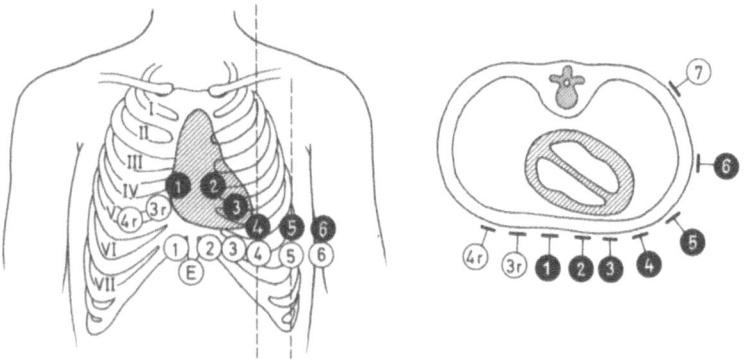

Fig. 12. Position of the precordial leads

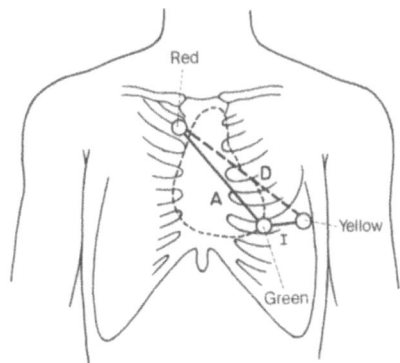

Fig. 13. Bipolar chest leads of Nehb

Esophageal leads are mainly of scientific interest. They are contraindicated in recent infarction, since reflexes during swallowing the probe may cause death.

All lead systems discussed so far have the disadvantage that their amplitudes are not comparable with each other, since the distance of the electrodes from the "heart center" and the intervening tissue resistances varies.

Physicists, mathematicians, and doctors designed a new system of leads to overcome these difficulties. Artificial resistors are placed between the individual electrodes and the heart center (zero potential) which are meant to permit comparison of amplitudes. *Orthogonal system of Frank*

The complicated switch panel is shown in Fig. 15.

Another advantage of orthogonal leads is the introduction of the sagittal plane for complete projection of all vectors of cardiac excitation.

As is seen from Fig. 16, the heart excitation vectors are projected on three planes. Lead $-x/+x$ roughly corresponds with standard lead I, lead $-y/+y$ with Goldberger lead aVF. The sagittal lead $-z/+z$ is new and roughly corresponds to the mirror image of chest lead V2 or Nehb lead I. x and z axis form the horizontal plane, y and z axis the sagittal, x and y axis the frontal plane. According to the so-called left-hand system (Fig. 17), the x axis is positively polarized on the left side of the patient if the observer points with his left hand (thumb of observer), to the patient standing in front of him, the y axis toward the feet of the patient (middle finger of the observer), and the z axis is at the back of the patient (observer's index finger). Division of the individual planes into sectors and degrees becomes clear from Fig. 18. Vectors that run ventrally or dorsally in the heart are particularly well projected on the sagittal plane. This is of advantage above all in infarcts affecting the posterior septum or the posterodiaphragmatic wall of the heart. *Left-hand system*

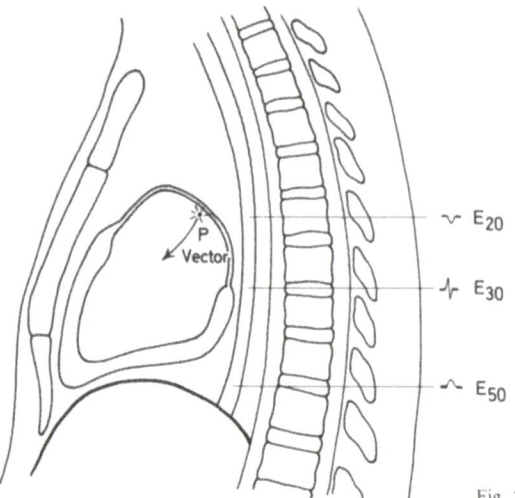

Fig. 14.   Esophageal leads

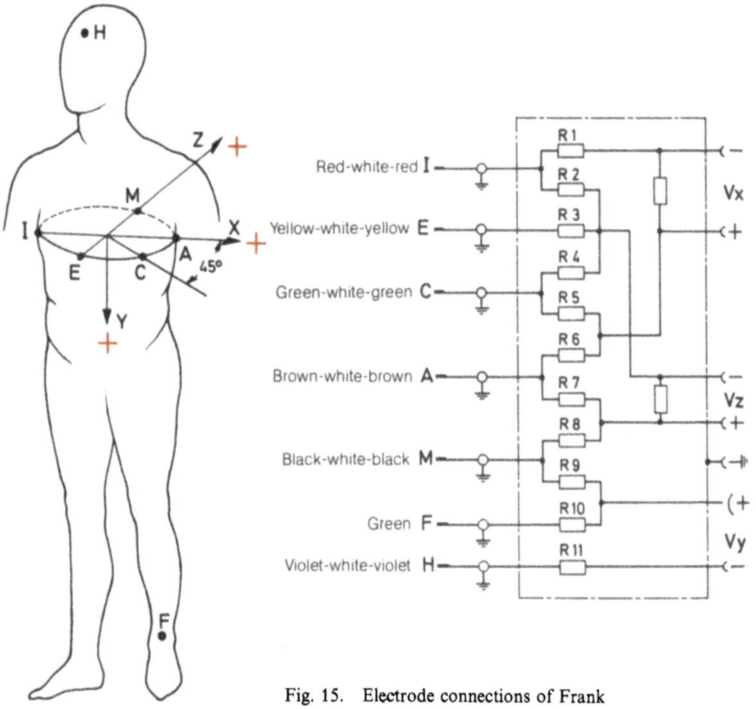

E_{20}

E_{30}

E_{50}

P
Vector

• H

Z
+

M

I

X
+

E   C

A
45°

Y
+

F

Red-white-red **I**

Yellow-white-yellow **E**

Green-white-green **C**

Brown-white-brown **A**

Black-white-black **M**

Green **F**

Violet-white-violet **H**

R 1
R 2
R 3
R 4
R 5
R 6
R 7
R 8
R 9
R10
R11

Vx

Vz

Vy

Fig. 15.   Electrode connections of Frank

16

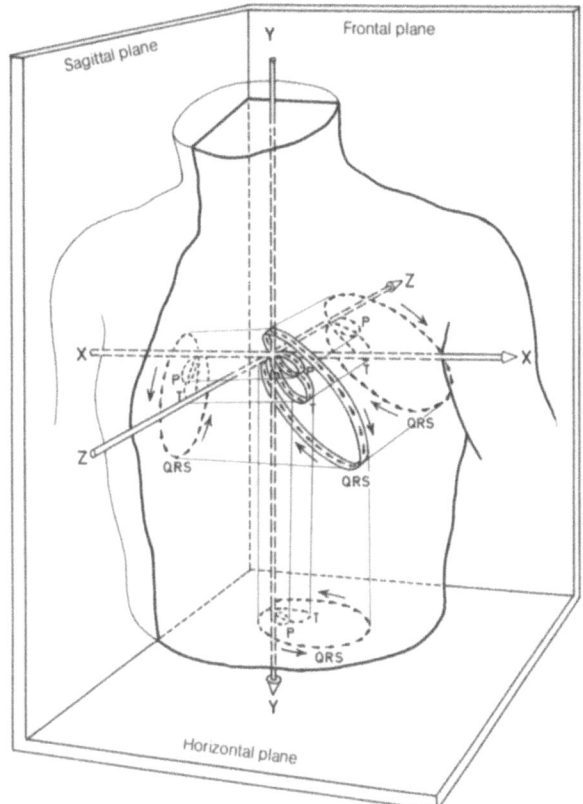

FFig. 16. Vector projection in 3 planes

Three leads are recorded with seven electrodes. This exceeds the information gained by the usual 12 standard-Goldberger and precordial (Wilson) leads, since they are complemented by the sagittal plane.

The electrodes are applied as shown in Fig. 19: electrode H is placed at the forehead or neck, electrode F to the left leg. The electrode for suppression of interference is applied to the right leg. Five electrodes are fastened around the thorax. They occupy a transverse plane, so-called dipole plane, marked by the point of contact at the 5th intercostal space with the sternum. This point must be carefully palpated and possibly marked. Electrode I lies in the right, electrode A in the left midaxillary line, electrode E in the anterior, and electrode M in the posterior median. Whereas electrode M is applied to the sitting patient, all other electrodes are attached to the recumbent patient. Electrode C lies over the palpated apex beat, in any case exactly halfway between electrodes E and A. The colored plugs of the Frank sockets of the ECG apparatus are connected with their respective electrodes.

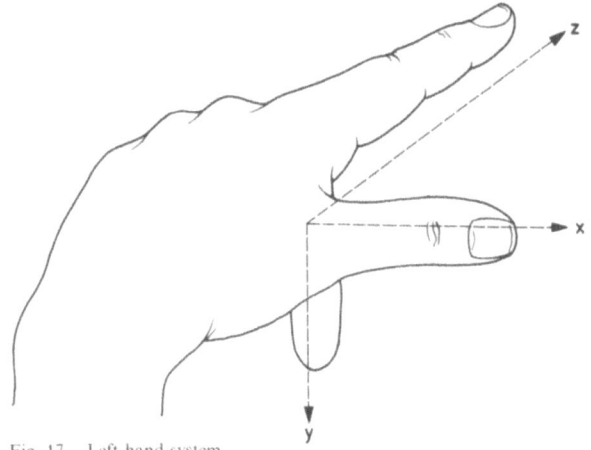

Fig. 17. Left-hand system

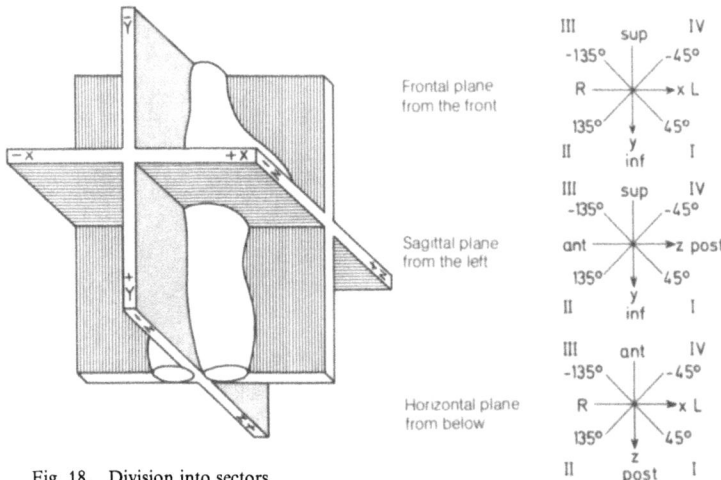

Frontal plane
from the front

Sagittal plane
from the left

Horizontal plane
from below

Fig. 18. Division into sectors

Since the amplitudes are comparable, they can be evaluated with the help of an electronic calculator. The "computerized" ECG serves to avoid many errors that arise from subjective assessment by one or several ECG interpreters.

Muscle fiber in the hexaxial system   Figure 20 shows on a model of a heart muscle fiber in the hexaxial system (circular scheme) mentioned above, how the respective vectors of the different leads or electrodes are seen. It should be recalled that the leads (I, VL) toward which the vector runs (electric axis), register positive waves, whereas those electrodes that face the negative terminus

18

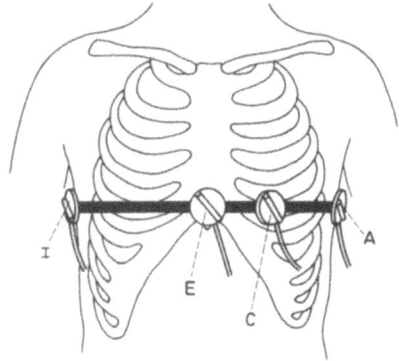

Fig. 19. Application of electrodes according to Frank

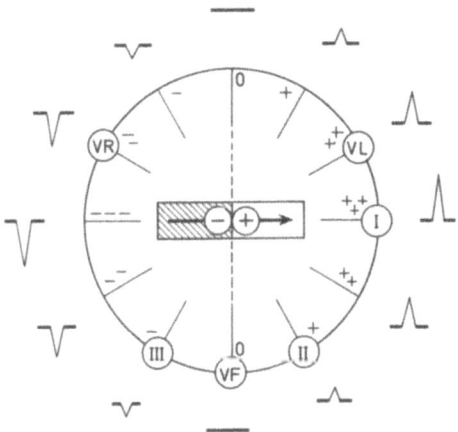

Fig. 20. Muscle fiber in hexaxial system

(III, VR), record negative waves. Leads perpendicular to vector direction, that is lie on the 0 isopotential line, do not indicate potential differences.

This is a good juncture at which to mention the chronological order of at least a few opposite partial vectors. Initially, the septum is excited from left to right during depolarization of the heart muscle. Only then is the main vector diverted from right to left due to excitation of the free ventricular wall. This sequence is simplified in the diagram (Fig. 21), where the septum f is first stimulated from left to right starting at point A, followed by the left ventricle with its thicker muscle f′ from right to left.

Partial vectors

19

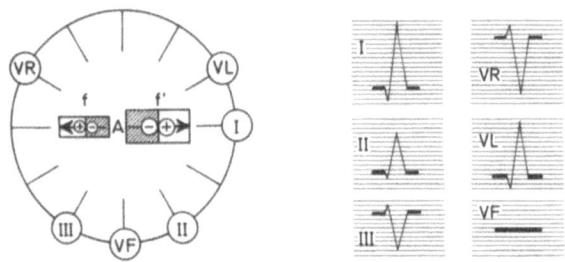

Fig. 21. Time sequence of activation of two differently sized muscle fibers

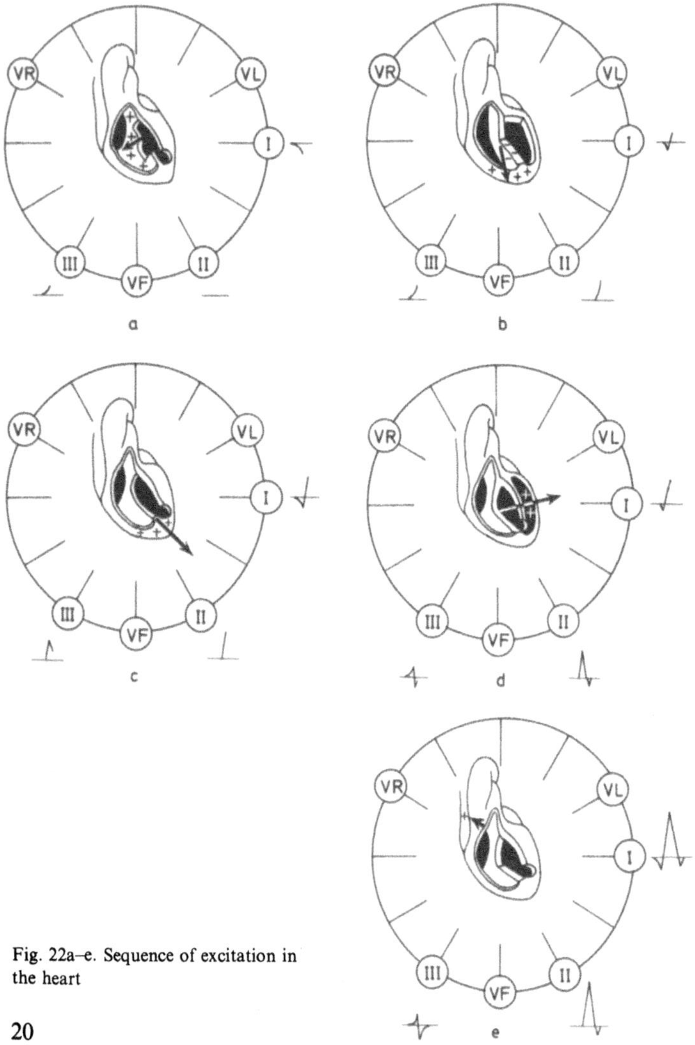

Fig. 22a–e. Sequence of excitation in the heart

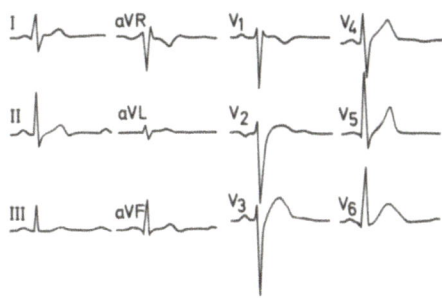

Fig. 23. (From Schweizer, W.: Einführung in die Kardiologie. Bern-Stuttgart-Wien: Huber 1972)

Figure 22a–e represents spatially the same process in the heart.

Figure 23 shows the ECG of a healthy young man. The various partial vectors will be analyzed on this at different moments of cardiac excitation.

In Figure 24 the projection of the integral vector is plotted on a frontal and horizontal plane after 0.04 s (R vector, red). If the vector is illuminated from the front, its shadow will be largest in the frontal plane in lead II, whereas if illuminated from above, the shadow of the spatial vector is projected onto lead V7. Since it is perpendicular on V4 in the horizontal plane, an isoelectric line, actually an equally high rs, will be recorded. In projection on the frontal plane it is perpendicular to aVL and thus produces a similar picture as in V4 in the horizontal plane.

In Fig. 25 all vectors of importance for the interpretation of an ECG

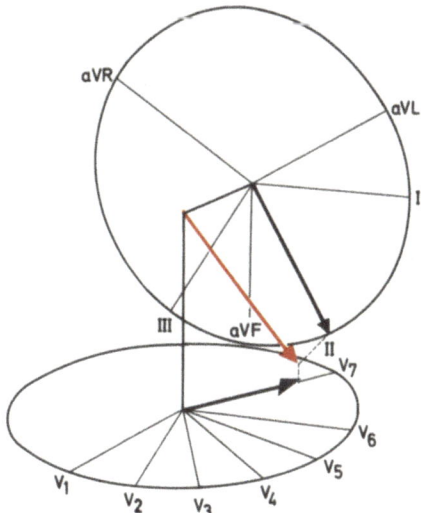

Fig. 24. (From Schweizer, W.: Einführung in die Kardio- logie. Bern-Stuttgart-Wien: Huber 1972)

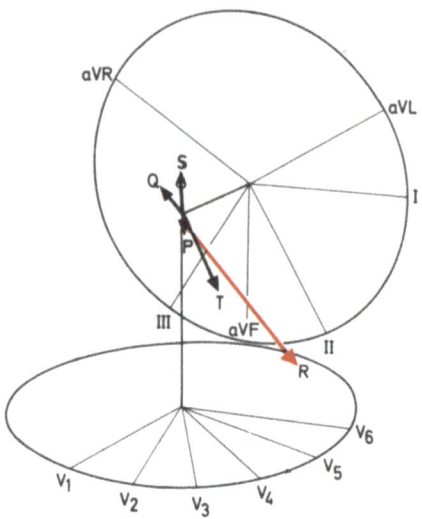

Fig. 25. (From Schweizer, W.: Einführung in die Kardiologie. Bern-Stuttgart-Wien: Huber 1972)

are concentrated. Illuminated from the front, their shadow projection falls unconstrained on the frontal plane; illuminated from above, their projection on the horizontal plane can easily be imagined. The vector bundle represents the most important sequential moment-to-moment summation vectors of atrial and ventricular depolarization, and ventricular repolarization (T vector).

Figure 23, 24, and 25 show the relation of the most important leads, still registered today, namely the interrelation of the bipolar Einthoven (standard), the unipolar Goldberger and Wilson (chest) leads, and thus give one a conception of spatial and chronological vectorial processes.

3. Interpretation of the "Electric" Axis of the Heart

The suspension of the heart by the large vessels at its base gives it its relatively great mobility. That in turn causes vectors to move in different directions.

Normally, the heart turns around the sagittal axis (Fig. 26 a); i. e., with a raised diaphragm to a transverse position and with descent of the diaphragm to a vertical position without abnormal changes necessarily being present. If a ventricle hypertrophies, its dominance can produce a similar deviation of the main ventricular vector. Left hypertrophy is usually, but not always, concomitant with a horizontal position, right hypertrophy with a vertical position of the vector. Whereas a transverse pattern disappears on inspiration due to depression of the diaphragm only when the heart lies transversely, it is preserved in hypertrophy of the left ventricle. Hence, an ECG in inspiration yields some information whether the changes are due to position or indicate hypertrophy. *Rotation around the sagittal axis* *ECG in inspiration*

The electric axis of the heart can already be determined from the ECG in the frontal plane (standard leads) and permits cautious conclusions to be drawn about the anatomic position of the heart's longitudinal axis. Although this is spatially not identical with the electric axis (integral vector), its projections frequently coincide in the frontal plane (see p. 26, Fig. 29 a, b). A condition for this is that the action current in the heart is normal and that the vectors are not displaced by a change in the spread of excitation in other directions that no longer correspond with the anatomic axis of the heart (e. g., bundle branch block).

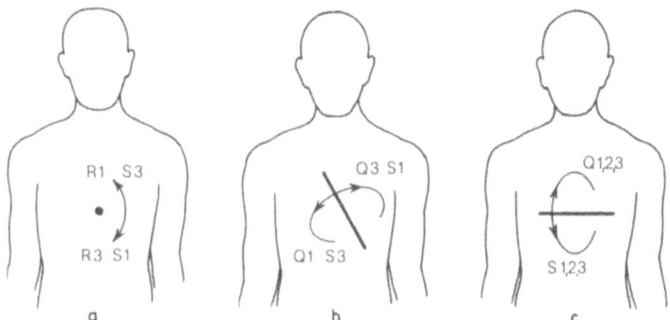

Fig. 26a–c. Rotation around sagittal, longitudinal, and transverse axes

The electric axis of the heart, by which is meant the rotation of the heart around a sagittal axis in the frontal plane, is defined from the wave patterns of the limb leads. The circular diagram (Fig. 20) is used again, remembering that all leads toward which the integral vector "moves" with its positive tip, record high positive deflections; whereas leads from which it retreats record deep negative ones. Leads that are perpendicular to the vector in theory do not register any potentials but in practice yield approximately equal positive and negative waves. The most important axis positions are shown in Fig. 27 a–e. The position of the integral vector can also be expressed in degrees of an angle. Alpha is the angle that includes projection of the vector onto the frontal plane with the horizontal. Normally, the main vector lies between $+30°$ and $+60°$ (intermediate axis, normal type). If it falls between $+30°$ and $0°$, a transverse position (horizontal type) obtains, whereas rotation beyond $0°$ to $-30°$ is called left axis deviation (left type). As vertical axis deviation (vertical type) is known a vector direction between $+60°$ and $+90°$, as right axis deviation (right type) with an angle from $+90°$ to $120°$. Extreme types of deviations to the left (anticlockwise) are beyond $-30°$ and to the right (clockwise) over $+120°$.

In order to determine the axis, the largest R wave of the limb leads is sought first. It is largest in the lead toward which the vector moves. For confirmation one looks for the lead with the smallest positive and negative deflection, i. e., the one to which the vector stands almost perpendicular. Finally, one locates the lead with the most negative deflection, i. e., the one facing the main vector.

As mentioned, hypertrophy of the left or right heart alters the heart position; thus left axis deviation is found in left hypertrophy and right axis deviation in right hypertrophy. However, it may happen that a juvenile of asthenic build may have left ventricular hypertrophy from aortic stenosis or incompetence but the vertical position of the electric axis may simulate right ventricular hypertrophy. Hence, precordial leads are essential in all situations where hypertrophy is suspected (see Chap. 8), since only they can provide more information on the localization of the hypertrophied ventricle.

Still more marked deviations of vector projections than those caused by hypertrophy are seen in hemiblock pictures (see Disorders of Ventricular Activation, p. 37).

Figures 28, 29c and d present the rotation of the heart around its longitudinal axis. It can be seen that the heart can rotate clockwise in the thorax, the left ventricle being displaced posteriorly. On the other hand, the heart can revolve anticlockwise so that the left ventricle moves more anteriorly. However, this movement is restricted (because the sternum acts as a barrier) and hence is less frequent. For the same reason rotation of the heart with left ventricular hypertrophy is clockwise more often than anticlockwise.

These rotations are already suggested by characteristic wave patterns in the standard limb leads.

If the heart revolves clockwise, the right ventricle will lie higher, the left lower. Thus, the main vector of the left ventricle moves away from lead I (also from aVL); contrariwise, the initial vector (septal excitation,

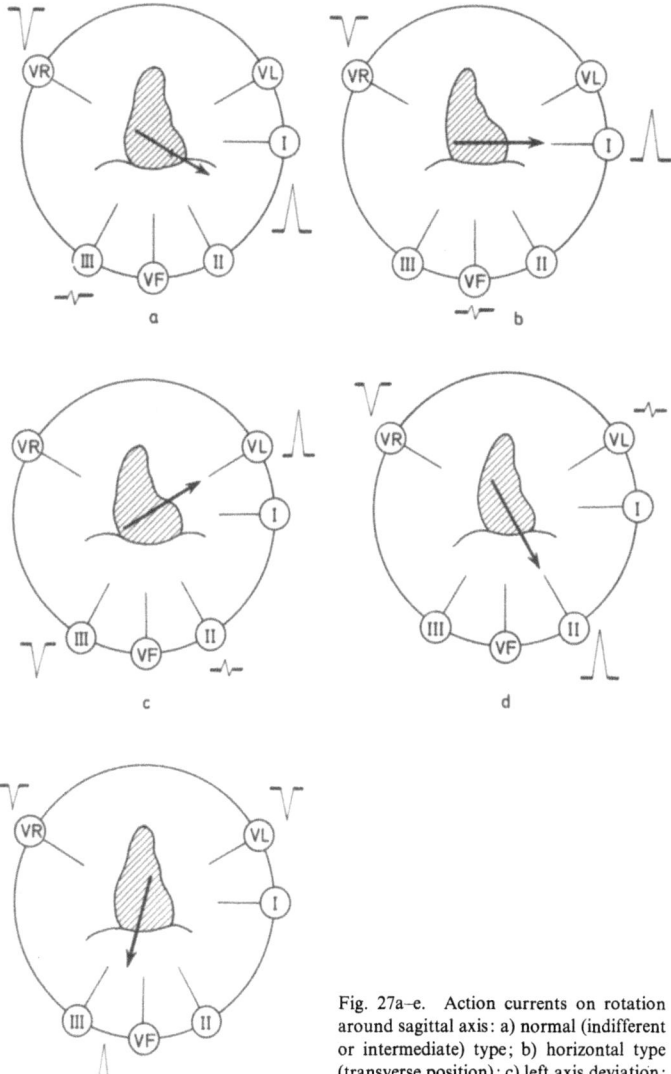

Fig. 27a–e. Action currents on rotation around sagittal axis: a) normal (indifferent or intermediate) type; b) horizontal type (transverse position); c) left axis deviation; d) vertical type; e) right axis deviation

25

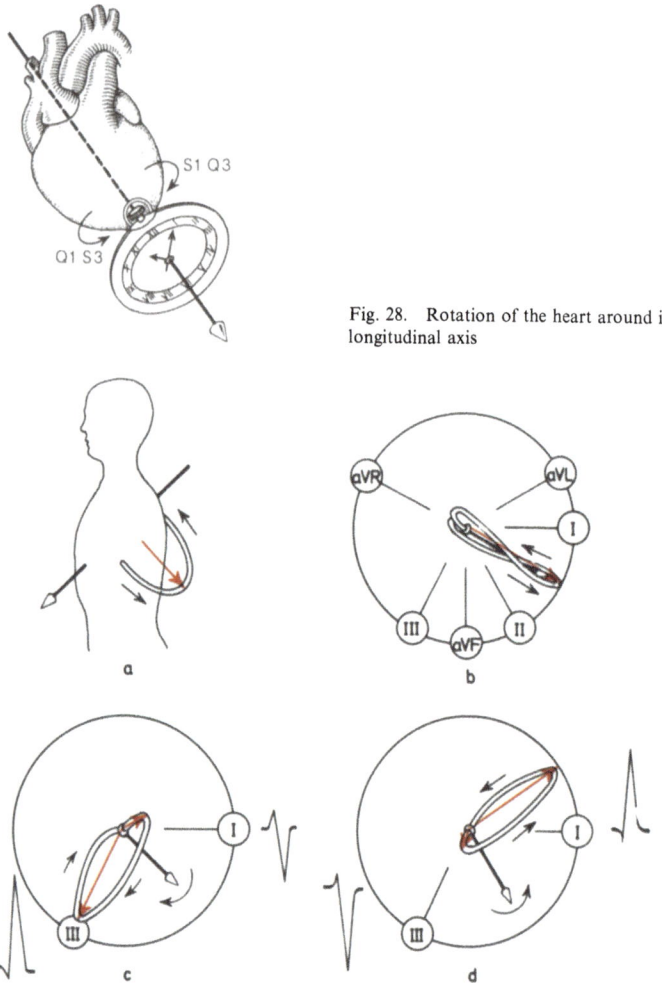

Fig. 28. Rotation of the heart around its longitudinal axis

Fig. 29. a) Anatomic longitudinal axis of the heart *(black arrow)* and spatial vector loop *(black loop.* Electric axis or main vector *red arrow);* b) its normal projection onto frontal plane (phantom turns toward observer); c) frontal projection of vector loop on clockwise rotation around longitudinal heart axis (S1Q3 type); d) frontal projection of vector loop on anticlockwise rotation around longitudinal heart axis (Q1S3 type)

Figs. 21 and 22 a) moves toward I (aVL). Therefore, rS is registered in these leads, but qR in III and aVF (Fig. 29 c).

The reverse is the case for wave patterns on anticlockwise rotation of the heart (left ventricle in front) (Fig. 29 d). Rotation around the longitudinal axis can also be demonstrated from the precordial leads.

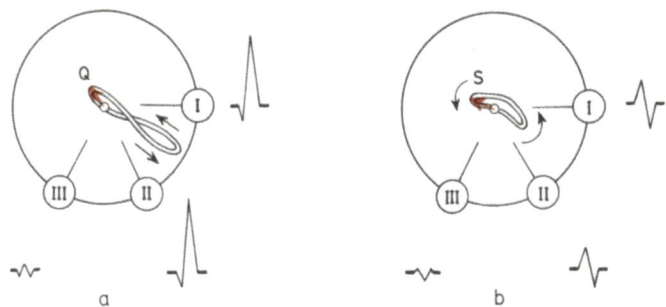

Fig. 30. a) Q1, 2, and 3 on anterior rotation of the heart around transverse axis; b) S1, 2, and 3 on posterior rotation of the heart around transverse axis

On clockwise rotation, the right ventricle affects a greater proportion of anterior chest leads. Thus, the transitional zone, where R and S have similar amplitudes, is displaced to the left beyond V4. This is seen in chronic cor pulmonale or emphysema. If the left ventricle revolves anteriorly, that is around the longitudinal axis in an anticlockwise direction, the transitional zone is shifted to the right, toward V3 and V2.

The heart, with its apex pointing anteriorly, can rotate around an imaginary transverse axis through the body (Fig. 26c). This only emphasizes the normal apex position; or the apex turns posteriorly into the thorax. On anterior rotation a Q is found in standard leads I, II, and III, due to the septal vectors moving from the frontal plane, and the frontal leads facing them; whereas on posterior rotation of the heart the late excitation of the left ventricle toward the apex runs posteriorly away from the frontal plane. Thus, S may be found in leads I, II, and III (Fig. 30 a and b).

Rotation of the heart around the transverse axis "Tilting window"

4. The Normal ECG

Figure 31 illustrates a normal ECG in which duration of waves and their amplitudes are plotted.

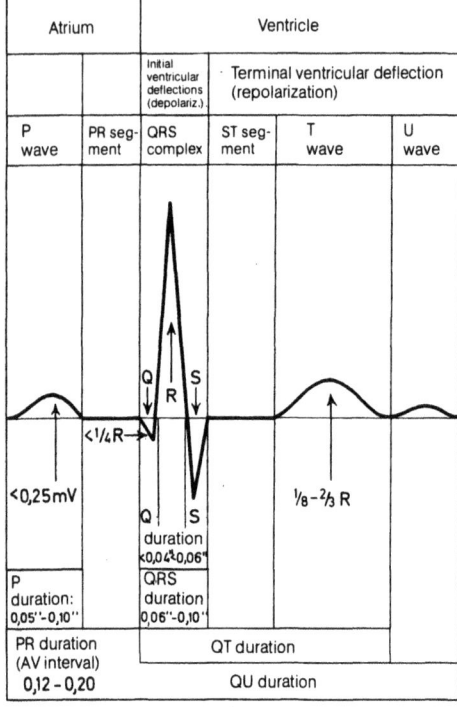

Atrium		Ventricle			
		Initial ventricular deflections (depolariz.)	Terminal ventricular deflection (repolarization)		
P wave	PR segment	QRS complex	ST segment	T wave	U wave
<0,25mV	<¼R→	Q R S		⅛-⅔ R	
		Q S duration <0,04²0,06"			
P duration: 0,05''-0,10''		QRS duration 0,06''-0,10''			
PR duration (AV interval) 0,12 - 0,20		QT duration			
		QU duration			

Fig. 31.   Normal ECG

4.1 The P Wave

Depolarization in the atria is registered as the P wave. Atrial repolarization is submerged in the ensuing ventricular complex; nor is it recognizable in the usual leads in total AV block. As mentioned, it is demonstrable on esophageal leads about 34 cm from the upper front teeth or via a central venous catheter. Duration of the P wave ought not to exceed 0.10 s in limb leads, 0.12 s in chest leads. The amplitude of the

P wave averages 0.1–0.3 mV, or 1–3 mm, if the calibration is 10 mm = 1 mV. Normally, P is positive in limb leads I, II, and III, and in aVL and aVF; it is most pronounced in II. It is always negative in aVR. Exceptionally, P may be negative in III, if the heart occupies a marked transverse position. Negative P waves also occur with taking the wrong electrodes, wrong electrode connections, situs inversus, or wandering pacemakers. P is always positive in left precordial leads, often biphasic (+ −) over the right chest wall.

Slight notching may be found in healthy subjects, even bifid P waves, due to asynchronism of atrial activation.

The shape is subject to considerable variation due to autonomic nervous system activity. If there is an increased sympathetic tone, the amplitude of P may increase above all in leads II, III, and aVF, and be mistaken for a pulmonary P wave (P pulmonale).

If there is an increased parasympathetic tone, P may become so flat in II, III, and aVF, that superficial inspection may suggest an AV rhythm.

4.2 The AV Interval (PQ or PR)

The atrioventricular conduction time, called the PR interval (regardless of whether there is an initial Q or R wave), should not be shorter than 0.12 s, nor longer than 0.20 s. It is measured from the start of the P wave to the start of the ventricular complex (QRS). With multiple channel recorders the "true" AV interval can be determined only by dropping a perpendicular onto the lead with the earliest onset of the P wave and the QRS, respectively. Prolonged AV conduction time at rest which becomes normal on exercise is not necessarily a sign of abnormality but is also found in trained persons with a high vagal tone. The PR interval is isoelectric, but may be downward if there are changes in atrial repolarization. In this case, the PR interval can no longer be used for fixing the isoelectric line — in comparison with which the ST segment will be elevated or depressed — but the TP segment will have to be employed. This is however not feasible in many tracings.

4.3 The QRS Complex

The ventricular complex (initial ventricular depolarization) usually comprises a Q, and R, and an S wave. Every positive wave is called R. The first negative wave preceding an R is always called Q, the first negative wave following R is always called S. A possible second or third R wave is called R' or R'' (Fig. 32). If several waves are present, it is preferable to speak of a split ventricular complex.

qRsR' qRsr' qrsR' qrsr'

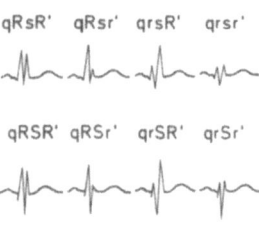

qRSR' qRSr' qrSR' qrSr'

Fig. 32. Notation of individual
waves of the ventricular complex

qRs   qRS   qrs   qrS

QRs   QRS   Qrs   QrS

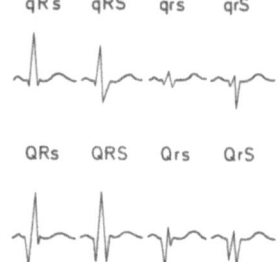

Fig. 33. Notation of wave amplitudes of the ventricular complex

Differentiation according to amplitude by using small or large letters is illustrated in Fig. 33; but there is no absolute measure for "small" or "large" waves. It is the relation of the waves to each other which is decisive.

4.3.1 QRS Amplitude

The amplitude of individual waves of the ventricular complex depends on the projection of its vector onto the plane of its respective lead. It varies with the axis. Hence, there are hardly any absolute limits for an amplitude still to be called "normal".

The amplitude depends not only on cardiac but also on extracardial factors. For instance, juveniles with a normal heart but a thin chest wall may have larger left precordial waves than elderly persons with left ventricular hypertrophy and emphysema. If the amplitude is extremely high, this is called "high voltage". The opposite is the so-called "low voltage" ECG; for this, fixed normal limits are available. The total QRS amplitude in limb leads should normally be no less than 0.5 mV (5 mm at a calibration of 1 mV = 10 mm), and in chest leads no less than 0.65 mV.

The magnitude of the R wave fluctuates greatly. In limb leads it averages 1 mV (0.6–1.6 mV), in chest leads of children and adolescents it may attain extreme values, up to 5 mV. The R amplitude increases from V1 to V4 in precordial leads and declines somewhat toward V5 and V6.

In contrast, the S wave (like the mirror image of a left precordial R), can often be very large in right precordial leads, as much as 2.5 mV (25 mm). Normally, S here is only up to 1.5 mV. S gains its greatest amplitude in V2 and decreases toward the left chest wall. It may be absent in V5 and V6. Its width should not exceed 0.08 s in precordial leads.

In the individual case the morphology of the Q wave may be important practically, especially in the differential diagnosis of infarction. The Q wave should not be wider than 0.04 s, otherwise an infarct should suspected.

However, the depth of the Q wave is not an absolutely reliable criterion, wheras its width can be of use in diagnosing an infarct. The normal Q wave may even reach 60% of the R amplitude in Goldberger's unipolar lead aVF.

4.3.2 QRS Duration

The total QRS duration is normally 0.10 s in limb- and up to 0.12 s in chest leads. In tall and muscular men it may attain 0.12 s also in the limb leads. QRS duration in excess of this suggests ventricular conduction disturbance. At times, the start and end of the QRS in a lead is so indistinct that a synchronously recorded second lead is required for definition (Fig. 34).

4.3.3 QR Interval (Intrinsicoid Deflection)

The instant the vector loop of the ventricular complex arrives at an exploring electrode and finally retreats from it corresponds to the moment when the upward movement (ascending R limb) reverses to a downward one (descending R limb). This is called the intrinsicoid deflection.

Synonyms for the intrinsicoid deflection are: arrival of negative potential, origin of greatest negative movement, QR(R′) interval. The interval from the onset of the ventricular complex to the appearance of the intrinsicoid deflection, the so-called QR interval, is measured on the isoelectric line from the start of the ventricular complex to the start of the steepest decline of the R or R′ wave, by projecting it perpendicularly onto the isoelectric line (Fig. 34).

Normally, the QR value in V1 is less than 0.03 s, in V6 less than 0.055 s. The difference: (QR interval left) minus (QR interval right) normally lies between 0.008 and 0.032 s. Prolongation of the QR interval indicates

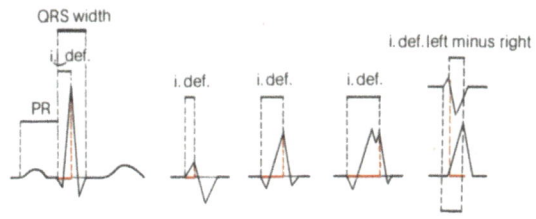

Fig. 34. Determination of intrinsicoid deflection

slow or irregular spread of the impulse in the ventricles. It can be determined for either ventricle separately and gains significance in the ECG diagnosis of "conduction delay", hypertrophy, and bundle branch block.

4.4 The ST-T Segment

The ST-T segment normally runs on the isoelectric line.

Depressions of 0.05 mV (0.5 mm) and elevations up to 0.1 mV (1 mm) are not definitely pathologic when they are left precordially. (In right precordial leads the elevation may even reach 0.25 mV = 2.5 mm.) An ascending depressed ST segment, that returning to the isoelectric line after half its total length, can be ignored in, for instance, tachycardia.

However, in patients suffering from coronary arteriosclerosis, flat ST depressions of more than 0.05 mV and running parallel with the isoelectric line, are not infrequent; these have to be considered as pathologic in conjunction with the clinical picture.

4.5 The T Wave

The T wave expresses repolarization of the heart muscle. Its amplitude must always be taken in relation to the R wave. Here also no absolute reliable criteria exist when the T wave should be called flat or still be regarded as normal. T is always positive in leads I and II, and approximately 1/4 to 1/3 of R, in left precordial leads at least 1/8 of R. T is always negative in aVR.

Children can have negative T waves in right precordial leads. In adults a negative T does not arouse suspicion when only in V1. Frontal projection of the vector of the T wave in adults should be no more than 60° from the QRS vector. Normally it is about 20° from the QRS vector (see p. 62, Fig. 55).

4.6 The QT Interval

This represents the total duration of the electric ventricular systole. It is measured from the beginning of the Q wave (if this is absent, from the beginning of the R wave) to the end of the T wave. Its duration depends on the heart rate.

Determination of the QT interval is difficult in hypokalemia, because a U wave may appear accompanied by increasing flattening of the T wave. The QU interval may then be measured in error for the QT interval.

4.7 The U Wave

The importance of the U wave is as yet not clear. Possibly it originates in an afterpotential during return of potassium ions into the muscle cell during diastole. If the T wave is indistinct or absent it must not be mistaken for it as can happen in hypokalemia. The U wave is most clearly positive over left leads, especially lead II. Negative U waves suggest ischemia or hypertrophy.

5. Memory Aid to Systematic ECG Description and Evaluation

A. Description

1. *Rhythm.* Regular or irregular?

   P waves: Do P waves follow each other regularly?

   Are all P waves identical? Normal or abnormal? (Check also V1.)

   Do identical ventricular complexes follow the P waves at identical intervals?

   Where does the main rhythm originate? (Sinus node, atrium, AV node, ventricles.)

   Type of main rhythm? (E. g., atrial fibrillation, atrial flutter, auricular tachycardia with block.)

   Premature beats? Origin? Escape beats?

2. *Heart rate.* The heart rate per minute is calculated on graph paper moving at 50 mm s^{-1} with divisions of 600/10 s ($=60$ s $= 1$ min) from the RR interval, obtained from the number of large squares lying between two R waves (1 large square $= 0.1$ s): Example: There are 10 large squares between 2 R waves, i.e., $600:10=60$ heart beats per minute.

   With a paper speed of 25 mm s^{-1}, the figures must be halved, not doubled.

   Our example: Five large squares lie between two R waves, i. e., $300:5 = 60$.

   State ventricular rate in atrial fibrillation!

3. *PR interval.* Measure where longest.

4. *QRS duration.* Measure where longest, and state where measured.

5. *QRS complexes.* Brief description, e.g., QRS I 0.11 s wide, QRS above 0.5 mV in height.

   Or: in which lead are Q waves wide or deep, R waves abnormally high, low, split, S waves deep, widened?

6. *Electric axis.* Comparison of main direction of QRS in leads I and III.

7. *RST segment.* Is the outset of ST elevated or depressed? How many mV? In what lead? Does ST ascend or descend?

8. *T waves.* In which leads are T waves flat, diphasic or negative?

   Is their direction opposite to the main direction of QRS?

   In what lead are T waves high, peaked?

   Symmetric or asymmetric?

9. *U wave.* Are U waves present? Positive or negative?

10. *Intrinsic deflection (QR interval).*
        In V 1 and V 6 normal or prolonged?

B. Findings, Summary, and Assessment
        E.g., atrial fibrillation, right ventricular hypertrophy, polytopic (multifocal) ventricular extrasystoles. Terminal deflection, as in digitalis.

C. Evaluation in Combination with Clinical Findings
        E.g., picture like mitral stenosis, digitalis overdosage?

D. Comparison with Previous ECG Findings
        E.g., compared with deteriorated, polytopic extrasystoles.

E. Suggestions
        E.g., advise daily check with standard leads after discontinuation of digitalis.

Request for ECG investigation:

Ward: ....

Name: .... Age: ....

Occupation: ....Date: .... Previous ECG: ....

Clinical diagnosis: .... Problem: ....

Subjective complaints from: .... Heart size and shape (X-ray): ....

Dyspnea, when? ....

Angina of effort: .... Abnormal thorax: ....

Myocardial infarct? When? ....

Blood pressure:.....Pulse: ....

· Vasomotor signs:.................................. Regular:....................Irregular: ....

Congestion: .... Goiter: ....

Lungs: .... Liver: .... Toxic:......................Obstructive: ....

Kidneys: .... Edema: .... Other: ....

Cyanosis: ....

Present therapy: 1. Digitalis or other glycoside. 2. Coronary dilators. 3. Procainamide, quinidine:

a) since when? .... b) how much? ....

....

Signature

Reg. No. ....Place and date ......

Name: .... Referred by ....

ECG findings: ....

Interpretation: (electrophysiologically) *) Tracing normal, at upper limits of normal, probably abnormal, certainly abnormal

Evaluation: (Only feasible if sufficient is known from the history and overall clinical findings. In discrepancy between ECG and clinical findings, the latter prevail.)

*) Underline as necessary

6. Ventricular Conduction Disorders — Bundle Branch Block

The right atrium is depolarized from the sinoatrial node craniocaudally, followed by the left atrium from right to left approximately 0.02 s later. Excitation (depolarization) travels along preferential pathways in the atria, in which an anterior, an intermediate, and a posterior bundle is distinguished in the right atrium, whereas a branch of the anterior bundle, the so-called Bachmann bundle, courses toward the left atrium. The three bundles come together at the atrioventricular (Aschoff-Tawara) node. Excitation slows here, but then rapidly passes along the main bundle toward the ventricles, where likewise three bundles (fascicles) are distinguished. On the left of the ventricular septum the left conduction system divides fan-like into an anterior and a posterior division (fascicle), whereas on the right of the septum, the right Tawara bundle (right fascicle or bundle branch) runs undivided. The anterior fascicle of the left Tawara system supplies the anterocranial portions of the left ventricle, the posterior fascicle the dorsobasal area of the left ventricle. Depolarization of the right ventricle occurs via the right Tawara bundle (Fig. 35).

The AV node, the bundle of His, and the left posterior division (fascicle) of the left bundle branch are supplied by the posterior

Normal depolarization

Atrial conducting system

Ventricular conducting system

Blood supply of the conducting system

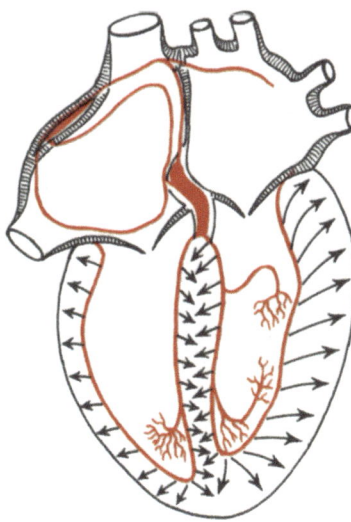

Fig. 35. Normal conduction system. *Arrows:* spread of depolarization in septum and free wall of ventricles

37

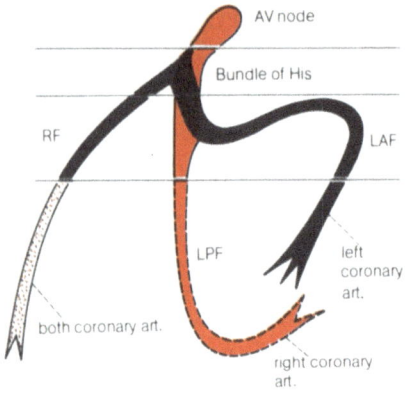

Fig. 36.   Blood supply of the conduction system. (From Schweizer, W.: Einführung in die Kardiologie. Bern-Stuttgart-Wien: Huber 1972)

descending branch of the right coronary artery in the majority of cases. The left anterior and the right bundle branch are supplied by the descending branch of the left coronary artery (ramus interventricularis anterior, RIVA). (Hence, this explains a bifascicular block in RIVA stenosis.) The terminal ramifications of the right bundle branch are supplied by either coronary artery (Fig. 36). It is not surprising that in posterior wall infarction, lesions are encountered in the AV node, bundle of His, and left posterior fascicle, whereas anterior wall infarction is frequently associated with a left anterior hemiblock, with or without right bundle branch block.

Each of the three divisions can depolarize its respective ventricle without delay. Simultaneous depolarization in both fascicles of the left bundle branch plays a decisive role in producing the normal ventricular vector, so that the integral vector is directed to the left, posterocaudally (R vector). Depolarization of the right bundle branch hardly affects the

Abnormal depolarization

QRS vector. But interruption of one of the two left divisions produces marked changes of the axis in the ECG. If conduction in the left anterior fascicle is interrupted, the left ventricle has to be supplied by the left posterior division; this causes an extreme left axis deviation of the QRS vector. Conversely, interruption of the left posterior fascicle leads to a right axis deviation. If all three divisions are interrupted, the picture is indistinguishable from a more cranial interruption in the conducting system. A picture of total AV block then occurs, independent of whether the interruption occurred in the AV node., bundle of His, or in the ventricle, by blockage of the three divisions (trifascicular block).

Classification of ventricular conduction disturbances
According to *morphology*
1. Unifascicular block
   Right bundle branch block (RBBB)

Left anterior hemiblock (LAH)
Left posterior hemiblock (LPH)
2. Bifascicular bundle branch block
Left bundle branch block (LBBB)
Left anterior hemiblock + right bundle branch block
Left posterior hemiblock + right bundle branch block
3. Trifascicular block
These correspond to a total AV block
According to *persistence*
1. Intermittent block: Delay or interruption of conduction is present only temporarily (e. g., in recent septal infarction or rheumatic inflammation)
2. Constant block: A Tawara bundle or peripheral portions of the conducting system are interrupted permanently (e. g., due to scars)
According to the *QRS duration*
1. Complete (total) bundle branch block
2. Incomplete (partial) bundle branch block
3. So-called hemiblock with hardly appreciable change in QRS duration
A bundle branch block is characterized by:

1. *Supraventricular origin of excitation.* With a caudal origin, distinction of ventricular extrasystoles is no longer feasible. "Supraventricular origin" means an impulse originating cranial to the bundle of His, that is, apart from the normal sinus rhythm, AV rhythm, atrial flutter and fibrillation. General characteristics

2. *Prolongation of QRS above 0.12 s* (in complete block). The entire depolarization is retarded due to the abnormal path of the spread of the impulse and hence QRS duration is prolonged.

3. *Prolongation of the QR interval over the left ventricle above 0.055, over the right ventricle above 0.03 s.*

4. *Secondary change in terminal deflection.* A change in depolarization elicits a corresponding change in repolarization.

5. *Prolongation of the QT interval* (electric systole); contrary to the WPW syndrome where it is normal.

6.1 Unifascicular Block

6.1.1 Right Bundle Branch Block (RBBB)

Complete right bundle branch block is characterized, as are all complete blocks, by a QRS duration above 0.12 s. The QR(R′) interval is 0.08 s or longer. In addition, right bundle branch block is divided into various subgroups according to typical morphology in right precordial leads and different axis deviations found in the limb leads. Special characteristics

6.1.1.1 Wilson Block

The so-called Wilson block (Figs. 37 and 38) is the commonest type of complete right bundle branch block. It is characterized by a narrow R wave in the left leads I, aVL, V5, and V6, followed by a frequently split S more than 0.06 s. An R or R′ wave is present in aVR. The T wave is concordant with the narrow R. The typical M shape of the main ventricular depolarization, with the deflection sequence rSR′ or RSR′, is seen in leads V1 and V2, or leads still further to the right. The second R wave (R′) usually exceeds the first in amplitude. The QR(R′) interval is 0.08 s or more.

6.1.1.2 "Classic" Right Bundle Branch Block with Right Axis Deviation

It is often called the "mirror image of complete left bundle branch block." In the right leads V1, V3r, V4r, but also in III and aVF, it usually shows a similar large, widened (low-amplitude) R as does left bundle

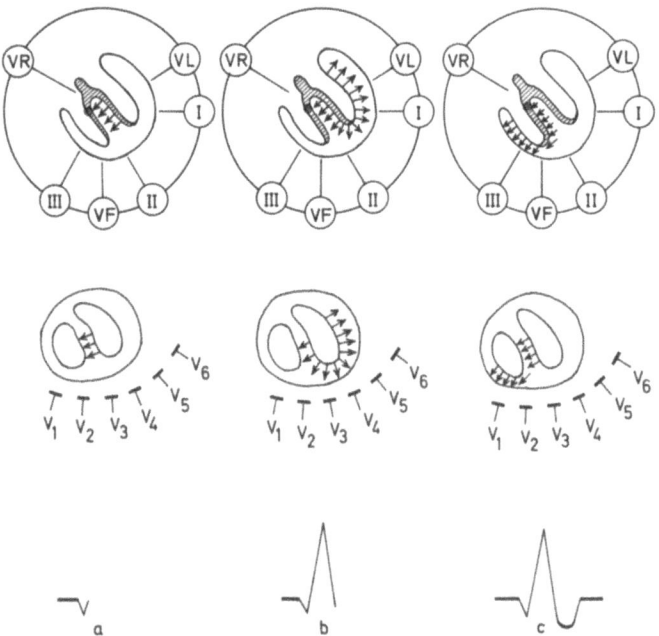

Fig. 37a–c.   Spread of depolarization in right bundle branch block. Example of tracings in I, aVL, V5–V6

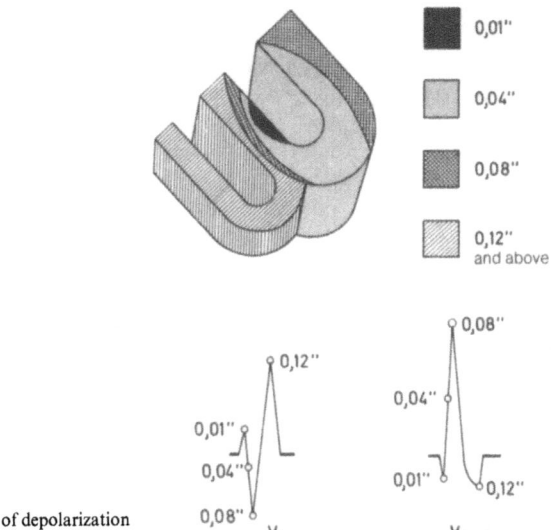

	0,01''
	0,04''
	0,08''
	0,12'' and above

Fig. 38. Spread of depolarization in right bundle branch block

branch block in the left leads V5 and V6. The comparison with a "broken-off sugar loaf" applies to this R pattern just as it does to the R of the left bundle branch block. In lead I r is followed by a large, often notched S of more than 0.06 s. Discordant to this S in I is a large R in III. QRS duration is also prolonged to more than 0.12 s, the QR interval is above 0.08 s. The repolarization is discordant to the main QRS deflection. There may be right or left axis deviation depending on the pattern.

6.1.1.3 "Classic" Right Bundle Branch Block with Sagittal Axis Deviation

This fulfills all criteria of complete right bundle branch block, but is distinguished by a concordant QRS complex with small and large, broad S waves in leads I to III. "Discordance" and "concordance" used in older literature depend on the projection of the electrical axis of the heart on the frontal plane.

The peculiar axis deviations of the two last-named types of right bundle branch block originate in an additional hemiblock or in changes of the anatomic axis of the heart. They are only encountered in organic disease, especially coronary arteriosclerosis. A Wilson block may occasionally be seen in clinically normal hearts.

41

6.1.1.4 Incomplete Right Bundle Branch Block

Incomplete types of block have a QRS duration of less than 0.12 s, the QR interval in incomplete right bundle branch block is above 0.03 s. There are subgroups also among incomplete forms of right bundle branch block.

Incomplete Wilson block (also called physiologic incomplete right bundle branch block): QRS prolonged to 0.11 s, slim tall R wave with a distinct S in leads I and II. In the right chest leads there is a typical RSr′ with r′ smaller than the preceding R. It is not advisable to call this variant physiologic incomplete right bundle branch block, since it may be encountered in cardiac patients. Observation of the patient is necessary.

Incomplete right bundle branch block due to volume or pressure overloading of the right ventricle: QRS duration 0.11–0.12 s. Right precordial rSR′ type. Preponderance of R′ over r.

Figure 39 reveals that similar RSR′ patterns can be distinguished only by vectorcardiography. For each case the projection of the loop of the vectorcardiogram onto the lead line of V1 is shown. In example (a) — cardiac dilatation — activation runs clockwise, and individual segments of the loop are projected onto V1 at different moments, with R′ having a greater amplitude, since the terminal part of the loop is larger than its first one. Example (b) — right bundle branch block — shows reversed activation, the loop being inscribed in anticlockwise direction. The

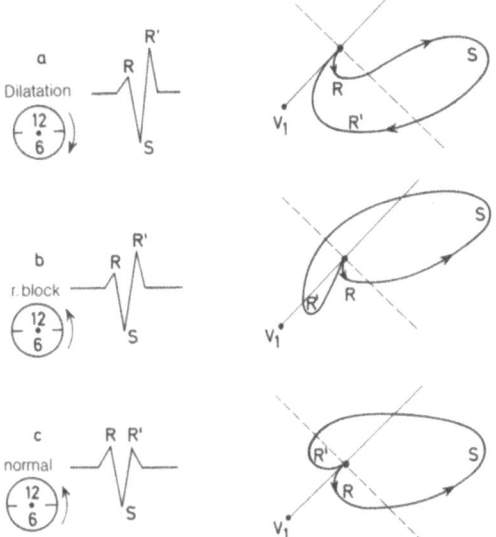

Fig. 39.   Differential diagnosis of incomplete right bundle branch block

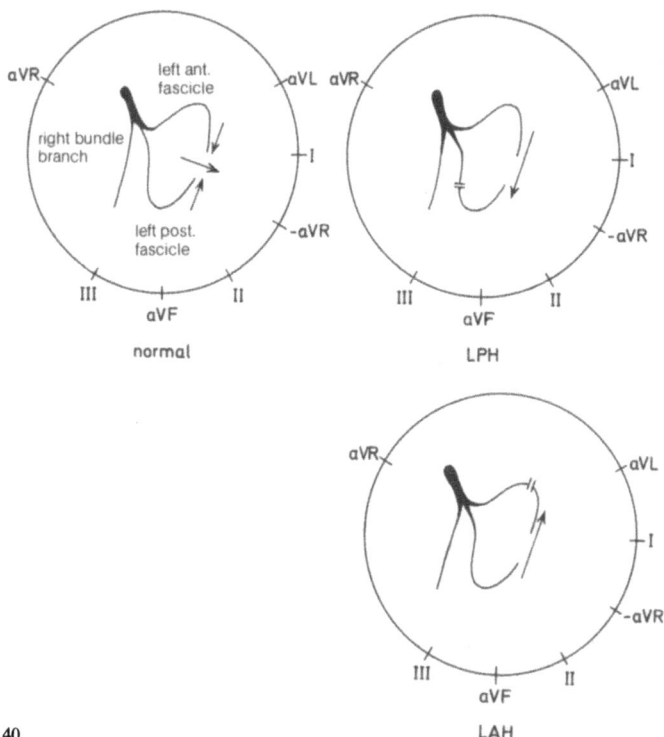

Fig. 40

conduction delay caused by the block in the right ventricle produces a terminal broadening of the vector loop towards electrode V1; thus, at that late moment, the summation vector projected onto lead V1 as R′ is greater than R. In example (c) a variant of the normal spread of activation is presented, the R and R′ projections onto V1 being about equal in size.

6.1.2 Left Anterior Hemiblock (LAH) (Fig. 40)

Interruption or gross conduction delay in the left anterior division (fascicle) leads to extreme left axis deviation with the axis more than $-30°$ in adults, or between $0°$ and $-30°$ in children. The ventricular complex is not definitely widened. Incomplete left bundle branch block will occur only if there is delay also in the left posterior division. Frequently there is not only a unifascicular left anterior hemiblock but also a combination with right bundle branch block; this is understandable in view of the common blood supply. This combined type of block is seen in anterior wall infarction with signs of occlusion in the anterior descending branch of the left coronary artery.

6.1.3 Left Posterior Hemiblock (LPH) (Fig. 40)

This is a rare type of block displaying right axis deviation with the axis between $+80°$ to $+120°$. This type of block, too, may be combined with a right bundle branch block. The hemiblock may be a sign of a posterior wall infarct, in view of the vascular supply to this region.

The hemiblock forms easily explain formerly misinterpreted axis deviations. Since septal excitation travels along an unaffected bundle Q waves are present in hemiblocks. Q waves are absent only on interruption of both left fascicles, since the septum can then no longer be activated from left to right.

6.2 Bifascicular Bundle Branch Block

6.2.1 Left Bundle Branch Block (LBBB)

Complete left bundle branch block (Figs. 41 and 42) QRS is prolonged beyond 0.12 s, the QR interval is prolonged to over 0.08 s. A broad R wave with a "slurred tip" is found in leads I, V5, and V6; Q does not usually precede it. Repolarization is discordant. The upward convex ST segment is followed by a ($-$ to $+$) biphasic T. Not infrequently the initial right precordial r is absent so that an anteroseptal infarct is mimicked.

In a complete left bundle branch block, both left fascicles of the conduction system are interrupted, a combination of left anterior and left posterior hemiblock results. The integral vector will take a direction between the extreme left axis deviation of left anterior hemiblock and the right axis deviation of left posterior hemiblock, i. e. the QRS vector is deviated leftward and posteriorly.

Incomplete left bundle branch block. QRS is not increased above 0.12 s, but the QR interval in V6 (V5) is retarded over 0.055 s. The ECG presents a "miniature" complete left bundle branch block. Small Q waves may precede R due to preservation of septal conduction from left to right. Thus, e. g. in left ventricular overload, say due to aortic stenosis, Q is interpreted as being due to septal hypertrophy. The essential reason for the persistence of the Q wave was mentioned above, namely that it consists of undisturbed septal excitation by the spared or at least better-conducting left fascicle. The appearance of an S wave after R in V5 and V6 in partial left bundle branch block suggests emphysema (clockwise rotation of the heart) or an additional right ventricular conduction defect.

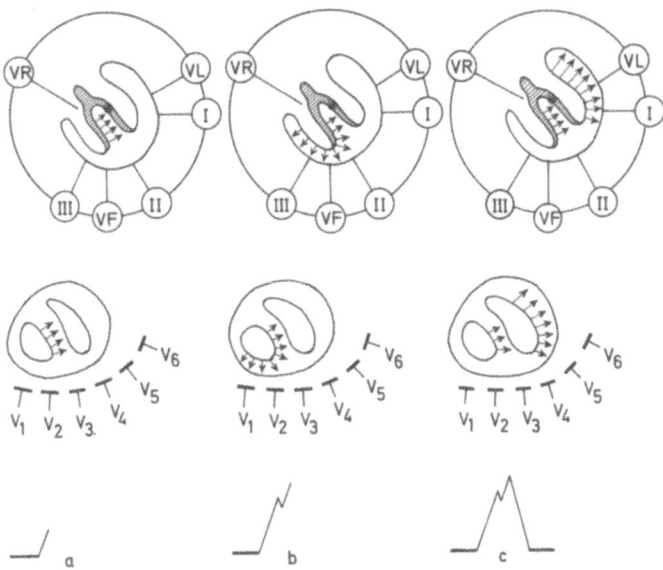

Fig. 41a–c. Spread of depolarization in left bundle branch block. Example of tracings in I, aVL, V5–6

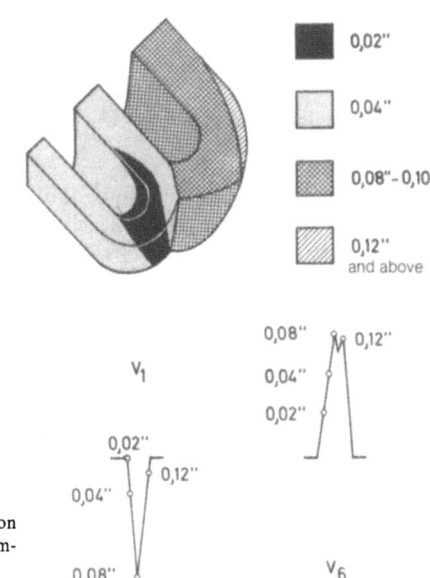

Fig. 42. Spread of depolarization in left bundle branch block. Example of tracings in V1 and V6

45

6.2.2 Left Anterior Hemiblock and Right Bundle Branch Block

Diagnosis of these bifascicular blocks arises from the extreme left axis deviation in standard and Goldberger leads combined with a right bundle branch block as RSR′ complex or broadened S waves over right precordial leads. Explanation of this pattern was difficult till recently, as it was not clear how the additional right bundle branch block arose in extreme left axis deviation, usually ascribed to left hypertrophy. As mentioned, this type of bifascicular bundle branch block frequently accompanies anterior wall infarcts.

6.2.3 Left Posterior Hemiblock and Right Bundle Branch Block

This combination is less frequent. It is associated with right axis deviation between +80° to +120° in standard and Goldberger leads, which is fairly consistent with a demonstrable right bundle branch block is precordial leads. Formerly these ECGs were thought to be due to right cardiac hypertrophy with bundle branch block. But this type of block is also observed in coronary arteriosclerosis without right hypertrophy. Complete so-called discordant right bundle branch block could thus be explained.

Figure 43 summarizes all described bifascicular blocks. It can be seen that a bifascicular block develops not only due to complete interruption but also due to delay of conduction in one bundle in conjunction with total interruption in a second bundle.

A few clinically important block tracings are exemplified in Fig. 44 a–d.

6.3 Trifascicular Blocks

These cannot be distinguished from total AV block in the ECG, since interruption between atria and ventricles is as complete as interruption in the AV node or the bundle of His. This type of bundle branch block is the only one that of necessity causes arrhythmia, since a tertiary

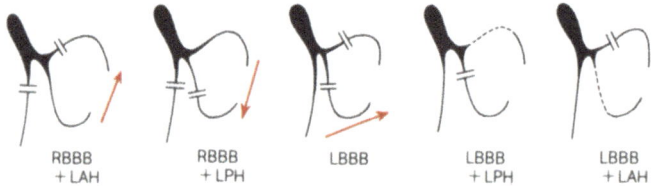

RBBB + LAH   RBBB + LPH   LBBB   LBBB + LPH   LBBB + LAH

Fig. 43. Bifascicular blocks

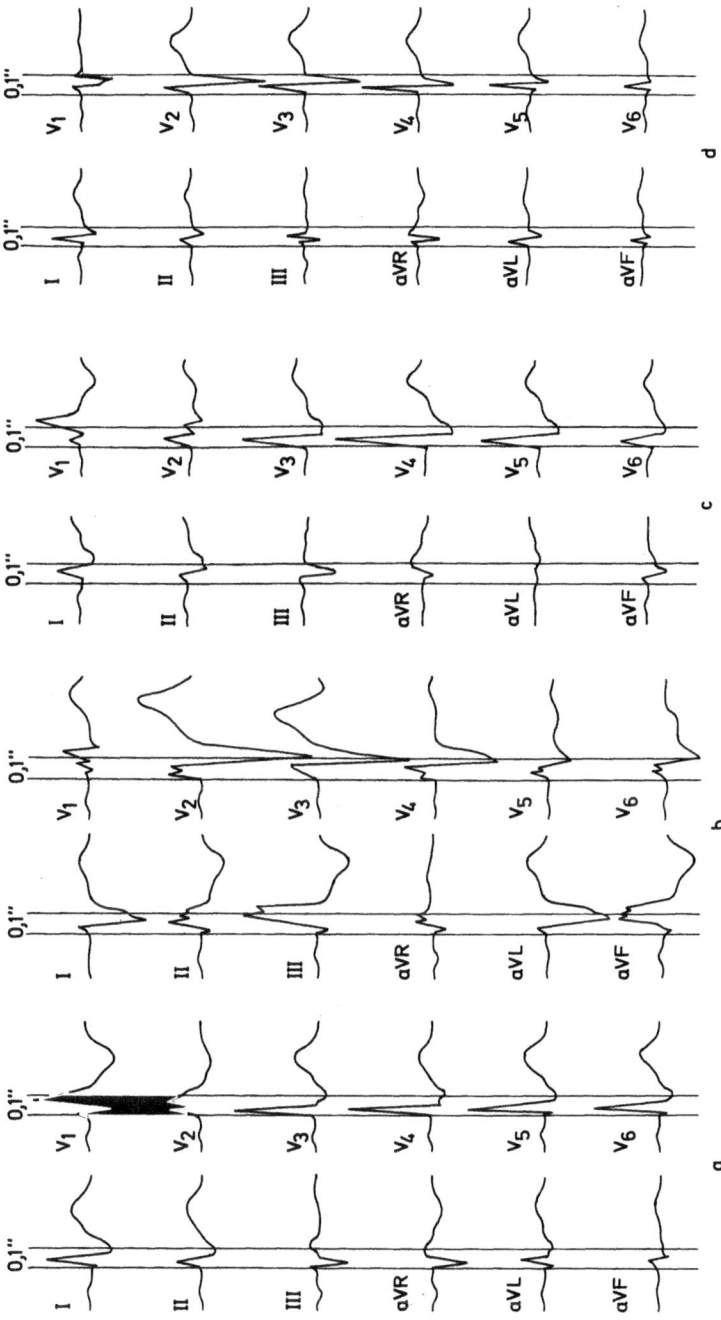

Fig. 44. a) Complete Wilson block; b) classic RBBB (discordant block); c) so-called concordant right bundle branch block. Differential diagnosis: left anterior hemiblock + right bundle branch block; d) incomplete Wilson block (so-called "physiologic" RBBB)

47

rhythmic center in the ventricle is forced to take over the pacemaker function (passive heterotopia).

Diagnosis of a hemiblock can be made from standard and Goldberger leads, whereas complete left and right bundle branch blocks are diagnosed with certainty only from precordial leads, for the heart axis is deceptive in the standard leads. Thus, on the one hand, in a complete left bundle branch block the main vector may be projected in the frontal plane at $-30°$, that is toward the aVL electrode, if the anatomic axis of the heart is markedly rotated to the left, as by left ventricular hypertrophy. On the other hand, with a vertical heart the same left bundle branch block vector can be directed toward lead II, that is toward $+60°$, in the frontal plane. However, in either case projection on the horizontal plane will not change. The vector can always be projected

Table 1. Classification of atrioventricular conduction disorders.

	ECG			His electrogram	
	Degree of block	PR interval	Ventricular complexes	PH interval	HV interval
Proximal AV conduction disorders	AV block I	Prolonged	Normal	Prolonged	Normal
	AV block II	Increased PR interval with occasional dropped systoles (Wenckebach periodicity, Mobitz I)	Normal, occasional dropped systole	Prolonged, occasional PH dissociation	Normal
	AV block III	No conduction	Normal	Interrupted	Substitute focus in bundle of His with normal HV interval
Distal AV conduction disorder	AV block I	Prolonged	Frequently lengthened (hemiblock or bundle branch block)	Normal	Prolonged
	AV block II	Mostly constantly prolonged, conduction occasionally interrupted (Mobitz II)	Frequently lengthened (hemiblock or bundle branch block)	Normal	Prolonged and occasionally interrupted
	AV block III	No conduction	Mostly lengthened (hemiblock or bundle branch block)	Normal	Interrupted

48

almost perpendicularly onto lead V4 in this case, and run toward the electrode position V7. Hence, it is recognized as classic left bundle branch block only in the precordial leads and must not be mistaken for a right bundle branch block, which could happen with an anatomically vertical heart axis.

Diagnosis of an intraventricular conduction defect becomes difficult if interruption is not of individual Tawara bundles, but due to additional or isolated conduction delay in the intraventricular bundles. In this case, AV blocks of first and second degree arise, which are known from proximal conduction disturbance in the AV node or the bundle of His. In Table 1 atrioventricular conduction disorders are classified in relation to these facts. The His electrogram mentioned in Table 1 will be discussed in Chapter 12.

In proximal AV conduction disorders the delay, or the temporary or permanent complete interruption, of conduction is located in the AV node or portions of the His bundle near the AV node. The ventricular complexes are not widened. In contrast, in distal AV conduction disorders, the interruption is localized in the ramification of the bundle of His into the three divisions (fascicles) or still further toward the ventricular chamber. A uniform, symmetric conduction delay in all three Tawara fascicles will not produce a total block but a first degree AV block, called distal AV block. If one of the fascicles is interrupted, and the other two are poor conductors, the conduction disturbance is asymmetric: either a left hemiblock or a right bundle branch block develops due to interruption of a fascicle; but a first-degree AV block still results from the conduction delay in the other fascicles. Second-degree distal AV block (Mobitz II) is in the majority of cases due to a trifascicular intraventricular conduction disorder. In any case, at least one fascicle has to be functional temporarily, since otherwise a permanent trifascicular, i.e., a total AV block would follow. It is this fascicle that determines the degree of the conduction failure. Distal AV blocks are therefore usually associated with bundle branch blocks.

Proximal and distal AV conduction disorders

7. The WPW Syndrome (Wolff-Parkinson-White Syndrome, Preexcitation Syndrome, Antesystolia, "False Bundle Branch Block")

The prototype of the WPW syndrome is characterized by two causally interrelated, abnormal properties of the ECG:

1. *Ventricular complexes with a prolonged initial deflection, mostly of sluggish start* and accompanied by more or less pronounced deformation of the ST-T segment.

2. *Shortened AV intervals,* since the duration of the initial ventricular activation is prolonged at the expense of the AV interval.

Another, not always present, associated feature of the syndrome is attacks of *paroxysmal tachycardia,* which occur in about 2/3 of the cases.

The ventricular complex is lengthened in the WPW syndrome, just as in "true" bundle branch block. But this prolongation of QRS is not at the expense of the ST-T segment, but of the PR interval, since the origin of the R wave is displaced in the direction of the P wave. The not infrequent result is a QRS duration in excess of 0.12 s and also a

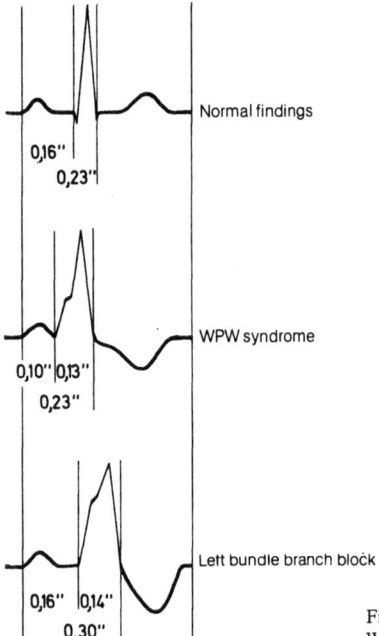

Fig. 45. Time relation of P and QRS in WPW syndrome and left bundle branch block

shortening of the PQ(R) or AV interval to less than 0.12 s. But the time from commencement of the P wave to the termination of QRS, the so-called PJ interval, remains unchanged. This point J (junction point) lies at the transition of the R or S wave to the ST segment at the end of the ventricular depolarization.

In bundle branch block, which rather resembles the WPW ECG except for the shortened PR interval, completion of ventricular excitation is retarded. But in the WPW syndrome it appears prematurely (antesystoly, pre–excitation). Hence, the AV interval is decreased by that time by which the ventricular complex is extended (Fig. 45).

The so-called delta shape of the R wave is notable. It results from an early deflection within the ascending limb of the R wave due to a

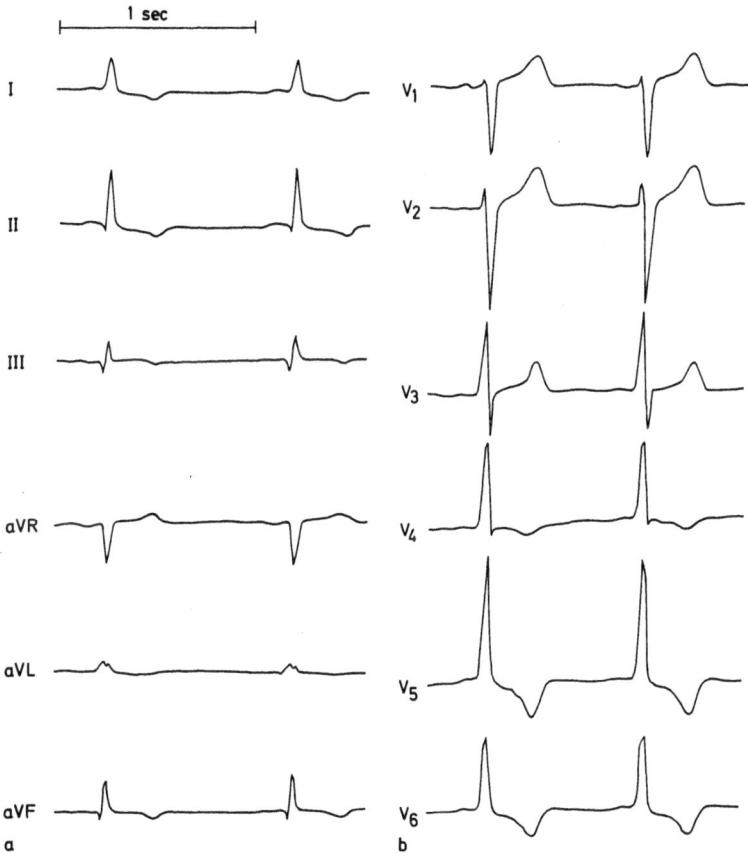

Fig. 46a, b. WPW syndrome Type B, so-called sternal negative type. PR interval 0.10 s. For another example see Fig. 68c. p. 84

premature depolarization of a circumscribed area of muscle in the ventricle. Thus, not only QRS duration but als QR interval are prolonged.

WPW types The following types are distinguished: Type A (left WPW): delta R wave over the whole chest = precordial positive type. Type B (right WPW): delta R wave in I, aVL, and V3 to V6 = precordial negative type. The typical picture of the repolarization in leads containing an R is characterized by an upward convex ST depression that continues in a predominantly negative T. Thus far, the pattern is largely that of a left bundle branch block, but the R wave mostly has a narrower peak in the WPW syndrome, whereas the genuine block displays a plateau R (slurred R). The less distinct the delta wave, the less the changes in the terminal deflection (Fig. 46).

Numerous transitions and variants exist in the same patient between the described findings and a normal QRS complex. The WPW syndrome may be constant or transient. The changes in the tracings can occur in bouts (intermittent, between normal deflections) or gradually. The alternating changes produce a "concertina effect." Thus, a delta wave may be prolonged spontaneously or transiently due to autonomic nervous system activity, e. g., carotid sinus pressure. Secondary changes in repolarization are associated with this.

Clinical evaluation Most subjects with a WPW syndrome appear to have normal hearts, but many tend to have paroxysmal tachycardia. "Harmlessness" of the syndrome can be demonstrated only by clinical and ECG checkups. On the other hand, the WPW syndrome can give rise to symptoms in inflammatory and degenerative myocardial disease.

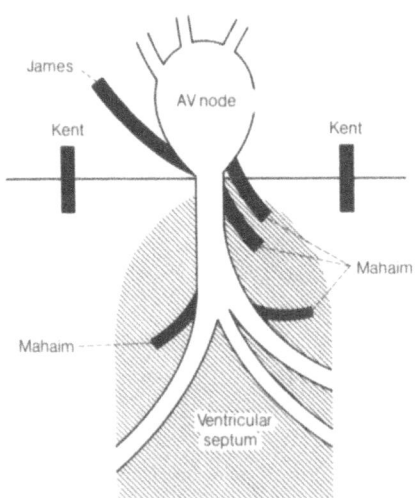

Fig. 47.
Paraspecific pathways

Preexcitation syndromes are caused by anomalous muscular connec- Etiology
tions between atria and ventricles, which lead to part of the ventricular
myocardium being activated prematurely. These "paraspecific" pathways are demonstrable as Kent's bundle between left atrium and left Kent's
ventricle, or right atrium and right ventricle. The former is responsible bundle
for type A, the latter for type B of the WPW syndrome. Other bundles,
the Mahaim bundles, have been described, which arise distally in the AV Mahaim's
node: the delaying action of the AV node is maintained and a normal bundle
PR interval with delta wave results. The so-called James bundle presents James's
a short circuit between atrium and distal AV node (Fig. 47). It causes a bundle
shortened PR interval but a normal ventricular complex (Lown–
Ganong–Levine syndrome). Finally, combination of a James with a
Mahaim bundle can lead to a short PR interval and delta wave (Fig. 48).
The James bundle is responsible for the short PR interval,, the Mahaim
bundle for the delta wave. Whereas the Kent bundle does not touch the
normal pathways of conduction, James and Mahaim bundles are
connected with the normal conducting system.

All three bundles may trigger retrograde excitation (reciprocal beats)
(Fig. 49, see also Re-entry mechanisms, p. 118).

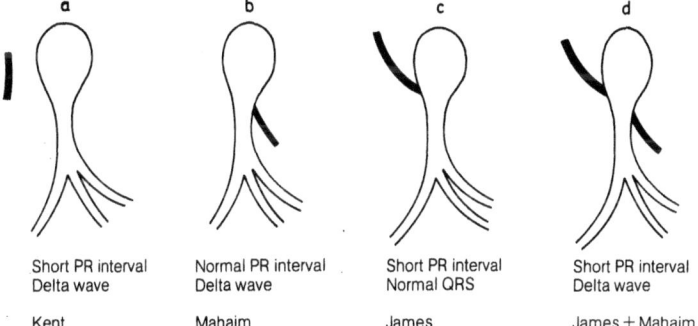

a	b	c	d
Short PR interval Delta wave	Normal PR interval Delta wave	Short PR interval Normal QRS	Short PR interval Delta wave
Kent	Mahaim	James	James + Mahaim

Fig. 48. ECG changes in different accessory conduction pathways

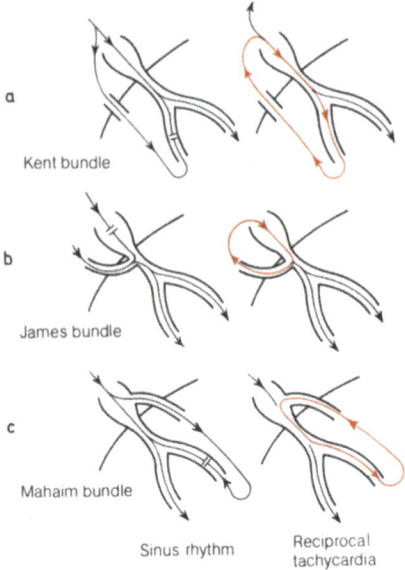

a

Kent bundle

b

James bundle

c

Mahaim bundle

Sinus rhythm   Reciprocal tachycardia

Fig. 49. Retrograde tachycardia via accessory and normal conduction pathways dependent on their refractoriness (see Fig. 89)

54

8. ECG in Hypertrophy of Individual Chambers of the Heart

8.1 ECG in Hypertrophy of the Atria

To begin with, the ECG of atrial hypertrophy will be discussed in detail, since its vectorial interpretation is easily understood and serves as a simplified model of the changes in ventricular hypertrophy.

Normally the atria are activated from the sinus node in such a manner that the right atrium is stimulated approx. 0.02–0.03 s before the left atrium. The main direction of the spread of excitation is from above downward due to the position of the right atrium. Therefore, the main vector during excitation of the right atrium is directed under normal conditions toward leads aVF and III. However, since the left atrial vector is directed rather toward lead I, the integral vector of both atria (the resultant of the parallelogram of forces of right-left atrium) is directed toward lead II, where the largest P wave can be expected on normal atrial depolarization (Fig. 50).

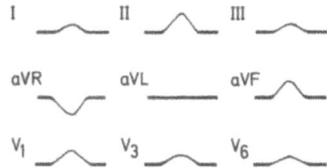

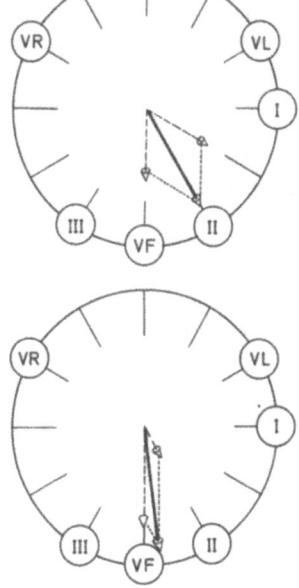

Fig. 50.   Normal atrial vector

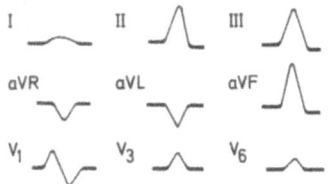

Fig. 51.   P pulmonale

55

If the right atrium hypertrophies, the right atrial vector running toward aVF will be increased due to the augmented muscle mass and the consequently raised potential difference, without appreciable change in the direction of the vector. The hypertrophied atrium enlarges downward and to both sides. As Fig. 51 shows, the vector of the right atrium predominates over the left. The integral vector, the resultant in the parallelogram of forces, is now no longer directed toward lead II but lead aVF. This large vector will lead to an increased amplitude of the P wave in leads aVF, II, and III. The abnormally tall and spiky P is called: P dextrocardiale, P dextroatriale, or P pulmonale. In leads II and III the amplitude of the wave is mostly above 0.2 mV (2 mm with a calibration: 1 mV = 10 mm). In lead I P is almost isoelectric, leads aVL and aVR face the tail end of the P vector and hence register a negative P.

What shape of P wave can be expected in the chest leads in hypertrophy of the right atrium? Basically the main direction of the P vector in the horizontal plane is directed anteriorly and slightly to the right. Hence, positive P waves would be expected in all precordial leads as for the normal heart, because the vector points at all the chest wall electrodes V1 to V6. Also, the P waves will increase in amplitude corresponding to the increase in vector. Figure 51 shows a diphasic P in V1. This is a P pulmonale in chronic cor pulmonale. Part of the right atrium lies below the plane of the lead due to the downward displacement of the diaphragm: the main vector of the right atrium first points to the electrode in V1, but will then pass by it toward the depressed diaphragm. Therefore, the electrode faces the tail of the vector in the second half of the atrial stimulation. Proof of the correctness of this interpretation is obtained in the heart of emphysematous patients by applying chest lead V1 a handbreadth lower, roughly level with the diaphragm, when only a positive P will be registrered. However, this biphasic P pulmonale is not widened in emphysema (in contradistinction to the biphasic P mitrale), but is frequently narrower than a normal P.

The main vector is directed from right to left, and slightly posteriorly and cranially, due to the position of the left atrium and impulse propagation originating in the sinus node, which lies at the junction of the superior cava with the right atrium. Thus, the head of the vector of the left atrium points toward I, aVL, V5, and V6, where corresponding positive waves are to be expected. However, since the left atrium is activated approx. 0.02–0.03 s *after* the right atrium, the P wave is formed chronologically by the right atrium first, followed by stimulation of the left atrium. Thus, the second part of P, i.e. the vector of the left, subsequently stimulated atrium, will be better formed in left leads. This difference becomes particularly distinct in marked hypertrophy of the left atrium. A bifid P develops due to the higher second (left) limb of the P wave. In addition, the whole P wave is broader and exceeds 0.1 s in limb leads and 0.12 s in chest leads.

56

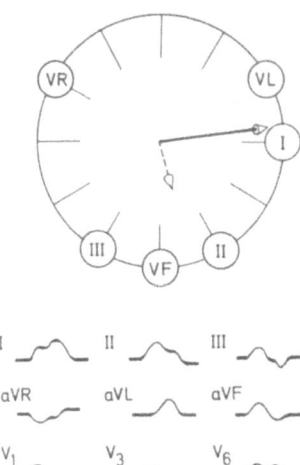

Fig. 52.   P mitrale

Figure 52 shows that in hypertrophy of the left atrium the vector is diverted mainly toward I, even beyond to aVL. Since activation in right and left atrium does not spread synchronously but successively, particularly in left atrial hypertrophy, depolarization in the right atrium, i. e. the main vector of the right atrium between II and aVF, is at least partly recognizable in the first segment of the P wave, and the vector of the left hypertrophied atrium in the second segment of the P wave. The axis angle of the summation vector of both atria is around 0°. This changed P wave is called: P sinistrocardiale, P sinistroatriale or P mitrale. Apart from the double-peaked, widened — and in the second portion occasionally raised — atrial waves in leads I, II, aVL, V5, and V6, a typical picture is observed over the right chest wall, particularly in V1: a small initial positive P deflection (right atrial portion), followed by a broad trough-shaped negative deflection. This is because the vector of the hypertrophied left atrium is directed away from V1 to the left.

In hypertrophy of both atria, P pulmonale and mitrale are found side by side. This is called "biatrial P". In leads I and II, P is tall and bifid, the second peak higher than the first and clearly widened. In lead III the P wave is usually diphasic, where the first, positive portion has a greater amplitude than in P mitrale. In precordial leads V1 and V2 — by which the atria are usually best assessed — a diphasic P is found, where the initial portion is high and pointed and the second portion negative depressed and broadened. Biatrial P

It should here be emphasized that P waves in particular are subject to functional effects. In cardiac surgery, e. g. during pericardectomy for constrictive pericarditis, P waves may within minutes display on continuous ECG registration variations from P mitrale to P pulmonale, although the anatomic substrate, i.e., the muscle mass of the atria, remains unchanged. Other factors play an important part, such as position of the heart and atria, nervous effects (in the orthostatic syndrome P waves become pointed and high in leads II and III, as in chronic cor pulmonale), and metabolic disorders. Changes in the P waves by themselves must never be overestimated in their clinical significance.

8.2 ECG in Hypertrophy of the Ventricles

In the last few years attempts have been made, following observations and investigations on the hemodynamics of congenital heart disease, to distinguish above all two types of hypertrophy. These derive from different hemodynamic conditions and possess, if isolated, specific ECG characteristics: resistance (or pressure) hypertrophy and volume hypertrophy (systolic and diastolic overloading).

Pressure and volume hypertrophy

Pressure hypertrophy develops when the ventricle has to eject against an outflow resistance (pressure or resistance overloading) in the circulation; e.g. the left ventricle in aortic stenosis, the right ventricle in pulmonary stenosis.

Volume hypertrophy develops when the heart has to eject a constantly increased volume (volume overloading). Aortic incompetence is an example for the left heart, atrial septal defect for the right heart (a permanently augmented blood volume flows into the right heart and hence into the pulmonary circulation due to the interatrial shunt).

Each of these two forms of ventricular hypertrophy is typified by an increase in amplitude of the QRS complex. In addition, in volume overloading (hypertrophy and dilatation) there is a simultaneous broadening of the QRS complex: a ventricular conduction defect is present (Fig. 53). For this reason the ECG of ventricular hypertrophy is discussed here, following ventricular conduction disorders (bundle branch blocks).

The ECG distinction of volume and pressure overloading did not prove as useful clinically as had been hoped. In advanced stages the ECG tracings in aortic stenosis and aortic incompetence may display similar changes, since in aortic stenosis, dilatation or ventricular conduction disorders occur secondarily due to chronic coronary insufficiency, and in aortic incompetence, repolarization irregularities occur, also due to coronary insufficiency.

But differentiation of pressure and volume overloading retains its value in congenital heart disease and in acquired valve disease (Fig. 54), if serial observation is feasible. Therefore, it should separately be discussed even in an introduction to ECG.

Our survey of ventricular hypertrophy (Tables 2 and 3) classifies

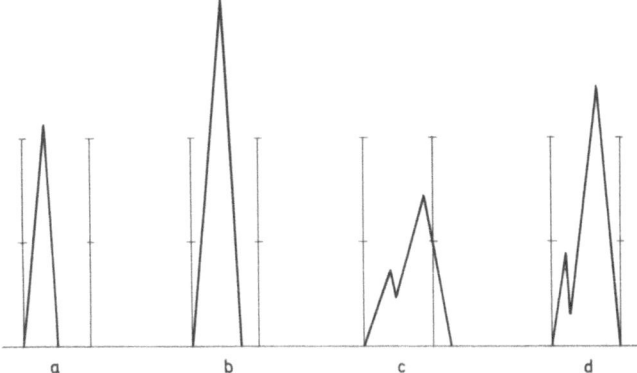

Fig. 53a–d. Diagram of depolarization in the heart as R wave: a) in the normal heart, b) in hypertrophy, c) in dilatation, d) in hypertrophy and dilatation of the heart muscle

possible changes not according to incidence but according to ECG "morphology". Not every hypertrophy causes changes that affect depolarization, repolarization and position at the same time, in the same manner and necessarily.

8.2.1 Depolarization
Size of Amplitude (Increase in Potential) (Tables 2 and 3)

Hypertrophy of a particular portion of the heart potentiates the respective R waves. In left hypertrophy they become larger on the left

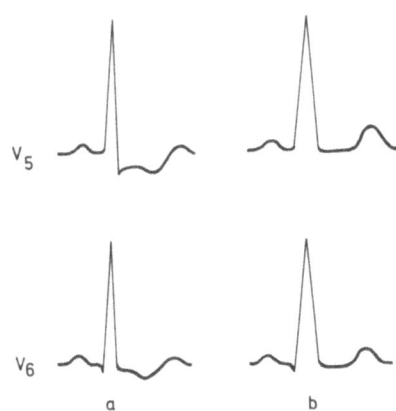

Fig. 54 a) Typical tracing in aortic stenosis (pressure overload): b) typical tracing in aortic incompetence (volume overload)

59

than normal; in right hypertrophy they increase on the right. "High voltage" is difficult to determine from a single examination, unless it has reached extremes and is obvious. The best aid is serial observation.

In principle all precordial leads should be included for evaluation, and waves measured both near the dominant ventricle and the opposite one. The greater the positive deflections of one side, the greater the negative deflections of the other. At times, only these negative waves (the corresponding S waves) are particularly large in the usual leads V1–V6; in this case they represent hypertrophy.

"Doubles" of high voltage

So-called "high voltage" ECG in the appropriate leads is caused not only by an increase in mass of heart segment (e. g., over the left chest in left-sided hypertrophy) but also the deflections are higher if the heart lies close to the respective leads, e. g. near the anterior chest wall in sparely built patients.

"Masking" of high voltage

Just as increased amplitude exists without hypertrophy, extracardiac effects, leading to low voltage, may prevent an increase in amplitude in common leads, even if hypertrophy is present, e. g., emphysema, effusion, scarring.

"Masking" and "doubles" are a reason why reliable indicators of hypertrophy cannot always be obtained from the QRS amplitude and from indices that are calculated from predominant deflections of the QRS complex in certain leads. The *index* of Sokolow and Lyon, calculated from chest leads, has proved most reliable in our hands. It is simple enough to provide orientation in general practice. Left ventricular hypertrophy can be assumed with a calibration deflection of 1 mV = 10 mm if the sum of the amplitudes of S in V1 (or V2 if this is larger) and the amplitude of R in V5 (or V6 if larger) is more than 35 mm (or 3.5 mV).

Sokolow index

The Sokolow index in suspected hypertrophy of the left ventricle:

$$S_{V1(2)} + R_{V5(6)} = \text{more than 3.5 mV}$$

(To be applied with reservation in young persons, as mentioned on p. 30.)

The Sokolow index in suspected hypertrophy of the right ventricle:

$$R_{V1(2)} + S_{V5(6)} = \text{more than 1.05 mV}$$

QRS duration and QR interval. Whereas an increase in amplitude of QRS may be the essential sign of any hypertrophy, the two other changes of depolarization (broadening of QRS and prolongation of QR interval) affect primarily only those types of hypertrophy which are associated with dilatation (volume overloading — eccentric hypertrophy).

As the diagram of impulse conduction shows (Fig. 53), the R wave in myocardial hypertrophy and dilatation is not only increased compared with normal but is also broadened. Indeed, pure dilatation of a segment of the heart also causes conduction delay in this area (widening of the

Table 2. ECG in hypertrophy of the left ventricle.

	Volume overloading	Pressure overloading
Depolarization		
Amplitude	"High voltage" of QRS: tall R in left precordial leads and in horizontal position of the heart, also in leads I and aVL; deep S in lead V2 and V3	
Ventricular conduction (QRS duration)	QRS duration in I around 0.10 s and above (delayed left pattern due to left bundle branch block)	QRS duration normal: 0.09 s
Arrival of negative potential (QR interval, I.D.)	QR interval in V5, V6 above 0.055 s	QR interval in V5 and V6 normal: up to 0.055 s
Repolarization	ST with notched transition to concordant positive T in aVL, I, V5, V6. Only in late stages does T becomes negative, as in pressure overloading	Roller coaster pattern (ST depression upward convex with − + diphasic T waves) in aVL, I, V5, V6. With increasing hypertrophy, opposite rotation of QRS and T vector
Heart axis (Direction of summation vector of QRS) Sagittal axis Longitudinal axis Transverse axis	Same direction but lesser rotations on all axes, as in pressure overloading	a) Moderate left deviation from normal position ($+30$ to $+60°$), in hypertension and old age: left axis deviation ($+30$ to $−30°$) b) At times, anticlockwise rotation (transition zone shortened and shifted to right). Extension of zone of large R waves to right c) At times q1, q2, q3

QRS complex) with diminution of registrable potentials (decreased amplitude of the wave). This picture of pure dilatation is observed clinically, e. g., in acute cor pulmonale.

8.2.2 Repolarization (Tables 2 and 3)

The characteristic change of the terminal deflection (hypertrophy repolarization, ST displacement, and T wave in the opposite direction (Fig. 55) to the typical waves of the QRS complex in the various leads, "roller coaster pattern") is encountered as an isolated sign, i. e., without QRS changes, particularly in conditions that require marked pressure effort by the ventricle and lead to concentric hypertrophy. It is debatable whether the cause is marked internal pressure or relative coronary insufficiency.

Repolarization in pressure overloading

When one follows the course of pressure overloading one finds that the T wave gets smaller in leads with a large R wave and finally becomes negative. At the same time, an

61

Table 3. ECG in hypertrophy of the right ventricle.

	Volume overloading	Pressure overloading
Depolarization Amplitude	Increasingly tall r or R' in V1–2, aVF, and III; deep S in V5–6, aVL, and I	
Ventricular conduction (QRS duration)	QRS duration in III around 0.10 s and above (delayed right pattern due to right bundle branch block)	QRS duration normal: 0.09 s
Arrival of negative potential (QR interval)	QR interval in V1, V2 above 0.03 s	QR interval in V1, V2 up to 0.03 s
Repolarization	ST with kinked transition to concordant positive T in III, aVF, V1–V3	Roller coaster pattern (upward convex ST depression with − + diphasic T waves). Typical finding in III, aVF, V1–3, but only when mass ratio right: left ventricle approximates to 1:1
Axis of the heart Sagittal axis Longitudinal axis Transverse axis	Same direction but lesser rotations (on all axes) as in resistance overloading	a) Vertical — right axis deviation (90–120°) b) Clockwise rotation, transitional zone shortened and shifted to left. Extension of the zone of large R waves to left. c) Apex rather toward back, S1, S2, S3 (sagittal type)

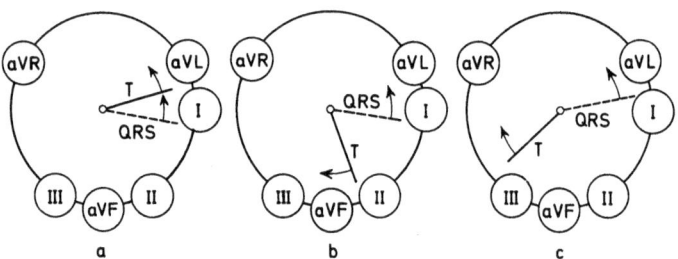

Fig. 55a–c. Diagrams illustrating relation of the T vector (——) to the ventricular vector (– – –). Normally the T vector lies to the left of the QRS vector. a) Still normal left axis deviation. Both vectors migrate in the same leftward direction in this purely positional abnormality. b) Moderate left ventricular hypertrophy. The T vector is displaced to the right and terminates on the right of the QRS vector. c) Marked left ventricular hypertrophy. The opposing displacement of the two vectors increases, hence discordant behavior of main and terminal deflection in the ECG

upward convex ST depression develops. It appears that the extent of hypertrophy and the degree of discordance of the R wave and the T wave correlate with each other. But a comparative morbid-anatomic and ECG study on 96 adults with aortic stenosis or left ventricular hypertrophy without myocardial infarct showed that an "extreme left axis deviation" (angle a less than $-30°$) was associated with a high incidence of myocardial fibrosis. Although the actual damage that could be blamed for the marked left axis deviation is not yet known with certainty, it does not seem to be the left ventricular hypertrophy by itself. Myocardial fibrosis must be assumed to be the decisive factor. Severe stenosis of the aortic valves is characterized by myocardial fibrosis just as much as by left ventricular hypertrophy.

For "doubles" of the negative T wave in an ECG of hypertrophy, see Chapter 10, Changes in the ST-T Segment.

"It is remarkable that diphasic T-wave change in eccentric left ventricular hypertrophy with volume overloading, uncomplicated aortic incompetence or ductus Botalli, occurs much less commonly and is often replaced by distinct high positive T waves in the left axillary region. The electrophysiology of this divergent behavior has not yet been elucidated." Repolarization in volume overloading

8.2.3 Position of the Cardiac Axis (Tables 2 and 3). (Direction of the Summation Vector of QRS and T)

It is generally true that the main QRS vector (the electric axis) is deviated to the side of the hypertrophied ventricle; not infrequently even more so than the anatomic axis. This deviation is the chief characteristic of the abnormal axis deviation: discordance of the preponderant waves in leads I and III (in addition: displacement opposite to the main deflections of the ST segment and development of the T waves).
Pathologic left type: tall RI, deep S III
Pathologic right type: deep S I, tall R III
"Doubles" of hypertrophy-induced axis deviation are: "Doubles" in axis deviation
  1. Anomalous position of the heart (e. g., dextroversion, simulation of left hypertrophy)
  2. Atrophy of the opposite side of the heart (e. g., extreme left deviation in tricuspid atresia, extreme degree of left hypertrophy)
  3. Conduction disorders (e. g., left bundle branch block in carditis)
  4. Infarcts

In theory, biventricular hypertrophy ought to be demonstrable by a summation of signs of left and right hypertrophy. In practice, recognition is rendered difficult in that the ECG picture of increased work of right and left ventricle is variably distinct. Here also serial observations provide the most reliable analysis. Bilateral hypertrophy

The most certain sign is an R : S ratio which increases both to the left and to the right. The lowest values are found in the center, or more to the right or the left, according to the dominance of the left or right ventricle. The supplementary leads V3r and V7 should regularly be obtained in addition to the usual leads V1 to V6 so that a greater field of recording is available to judge the R : S ratio.

The QR interval over the right ventricle increases, i. e., the difference between the QR interval in V5 and V1 becomes smaller.

The T waves, which in left ventricular hypertrophy due to essential hypertension, for example, are initially negative only over the left precordium, become negative parasternally as well in overloading of the right heart.

Rotation about the sagittal axis. Increasing vertical axis deviation, i. e., the summation vector of QRS is rotated from about 0° to +60° or beyond.

Rotation about the longitudinal axis. The junctional zone is displaced to the left.

P wave. P mitrale changes to P biatriale.

On sudden right overloading, e. g., due to acute cor pulmonale after pulmonary embolism, the signs just mentioned develop within hours.

Typical ECG in mitral stenosis (serial observation)   The course of mitral stenosis will be discussed at the end of this chapter, as a typical model of combined ECG signs in hypertrophy of individual segments of the heart. This most common rheumatic valvar defect is one of the few cardiac diseases in which a tentative diagnosis may be made from the ECG alone, because of a typical combination of ECG signs of hypertrophy of the left atrium and the right ventricle.

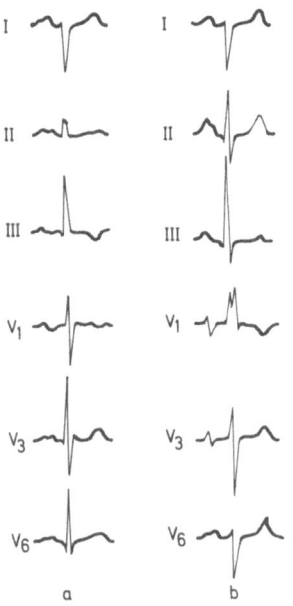

Fig. 56. Serial observation of course in mitral stenosis

Figure 56a presents diagrammatically the ECG pattern of pure mitral stenosis in a relatively early stage.

1. P mitrale.

(Atrial vector around 0°, bifid broad P in leads I and II, and V5, diphasic P with predominantly negative phase in V1).

2. Vertical position of the QRS vector in frontal projection: angle a more than $+90°$.

(The higher the pressure in the right chamber, the greater the axis deviation to the right.)

3. Signs of right ventricular hypertrophy in precordial leads not yet definite.

Figure 56b is a diagram of the ECG pattern in pure mitral stenosis of a late stage.

1. P biatriale (biatrial P).

(P mitrale and P pulmonale, angle a of the atrial vector about $+60°$, double peak most distinct in lead II, positive phase of P in V1 more marked than the negative phase.)

2. Right deviation of the QRS vector still more marked than in a (angle a more than 120°).

3. Amplitude of R in lead III higher than in (a).

4. Signs of ventricular hypertrophy in precordial leads (tall broad R in V1, S in V5, abnormal ST in V1, as in concentric hypertrophy).

Table 4. Synopsis of clinical and ECG findings in mitral stenosis

Severity	Complaints	PCP mean mmHg	Pulm. art. P_s mmHg	ECG	MOT ms	Opening area cm²
I	None	< 12	< 30	SR, maybe P mitrale	> 90	< 4
II	With marked over-loading	12–20	30–50	SR, mitral P	70–90	> 1.5
III	With mild overloa-ding	21–30	51–80	Atrial fibr., slight RV hyper-trophy	60–70	1.5–0.5
IV	At rest	> 30	> 80	Atrial fibr., marked RV hyper-trophy	< 60	< 0.5

Abbreviations used in Table 4: PCP, pulmonary capillary pressure: P_s, pulmonary systolic pressure: MOT, mitral opening time; SR, sinus rhythm; fibr., fibrillation; RV, right ventricle

5. In pure mitral stenosis no changes in repolarization suggesting myocardial damage or disordered blood supply are to be expected in left ventricular leads. They are absent also in examples (a) and (b). (If they do occur either co-existing mitral incompetence or myocardial fibrosis has to be considered.) The subjective and objective parameters listed in Table 4 should be consulted for assessment of the severity of mitral stenosis.

9. ECG in Myocardial Infarction

Hypotheses of necrosis, injury, ischemia
ECG in necrosis (Q in infarction)
ECG in injury (changes in outer layers — ST elevation; subepicardial
 type)
ECG in ischemia (negative terminal T)
ECG in chronic, general hypoxia (alteration of inner layers — ST
 depression; subendocardial type)
ECG in acute hypoxia (wide positive "asphyxial" T)
Site of infarct
Development and stages of infarction
Differential diagnosis of infarction
Infarction and bundle branch block

9.1 Hypotheses of Necrosis, Injury, Ischemia

Typical ECG changes in myocardial infarction
   1. Of the ventricular complex: necrosis Q or QS
   2. Of the ST segment: ST elevation due to changes in outer layers
   3. Of the T wave: negative terminal symmetry
   Below the attempt will be made to clarify these changes uniformly by
vectorial interpretation. It remains an open question as to how far these
hypotheses hold true.

9.1.1 ECG in Necrosis (Q in Infarction)

Under normal conditions the initial vectors of ventricular depolarization are produced within the first 0.04 s by electromotor forces in the
subendocardial layers of septum and free wall of the left ventricle. They
all turn away from the interior of the ventricle. The resultant of these
initial partial vectors is more or less parallel to the summation vector of
the whole ventricular complex: to the left downward and backward, as
Fig. 57 shows.
   If necrotic tissues after infarction prevent electric forces from being
produced in the first 0.04 s of the QRS duration, only the vectors of the
healthy segments of the ventricles remain. Therefore, their summation
vector will be directed away from the infarcted area. Deep and wide Q
waves will appear on the frontal (limb leads) or the horizontal plane

(chest leads), according to the projection of this initial vector. In transmural anterior wall infarction completely negative, i. e., QS, complexes will be found in those chest leads which lie directly over the infarct.

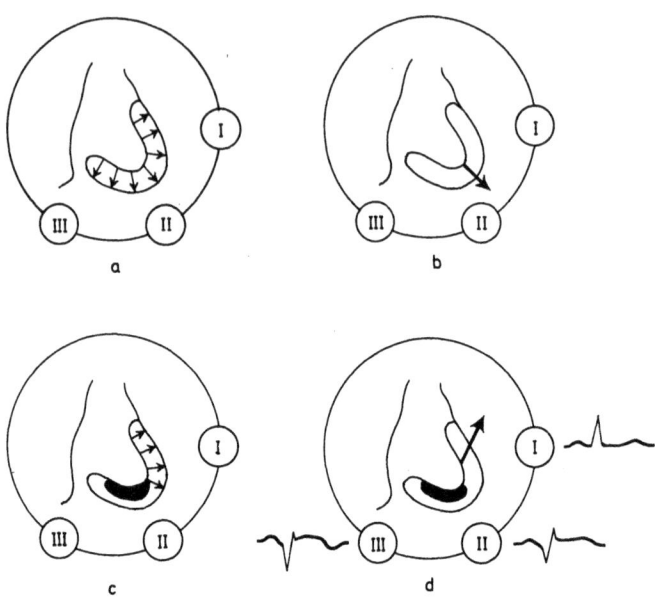

a　　　　　　　　b

c　　　　　　　　d

Fig. 57a–d. Initial vectors in normal spread of conduction (a, b) and in posterior wall infarction (c, d)

9.1.2 ECG in Injury (Changes in Outer Layers – ST Elevation)

In coronary artery occlusion, severe metabolic disturbances with inflammatory reaction occur mainly subepicardially, in the immediate surroundings of the necrotic area. This is called electrophysiologically a "zone of injury". If conduction is affected in this area (e. g., in infarction pericarditis), the outer layers are less "well" depolarized, i. e., less electronegative, at the end of the depolarization (at the termination of the ventricular complex) than the inner layers of the myocardium. Thus, a potential difference arises from this at the end of depolarization, i. e., a vector at the time of the ST-T segment where normally there are no potential differences This is a vector which is directed from within outward, toward the relatively electropositive or less negative areas (Fig. 58). For this reason a positive deflection is to be expected, i. e., an elevation of the ST-T segment, in all leads toward which this vector is directed. The highest ST elevation will be expected in those leads that form the smallest angle with the abnormal summation vector. (In the example in Fig. 58, lead II in the frontal plane, V4 in the horizontal plane).

In summary, the ST vector in transmural or subepicardial (outer layer) changes is directed toward the zone of the injury.

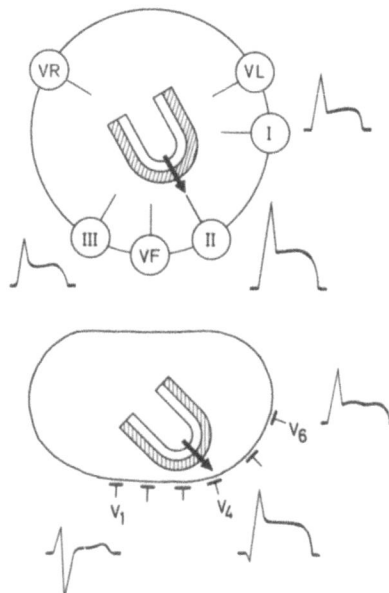

Fig. 58. ST vector in changes
of the outer layers

9.1.3 ECG in Local Ischemia (Negative Terminal T)

The main T vector is directed away from the site of the infarction and more or less parallel to the initial (0.04 s) vector.

How is a negative terminal T wave to be interpreted vectorially in ischemia? Several hypotheses and considerations have been proffered. The outer layers are still electronegative, whereas the inner layers are fully repolarized again and are electropositive. In the phase of repolarization, a vector will be directed from without inward, since the vector head always points toward the region of greatest electropositivity.

In coronary insufficiency the inner layers of the myocardium are probably less excitable (depolarizable) and hence display less electronegativity at the end of depolarization. Therefore, repolarization in these subendocardial muscle layers can be concluded sooner than in the outer layers.

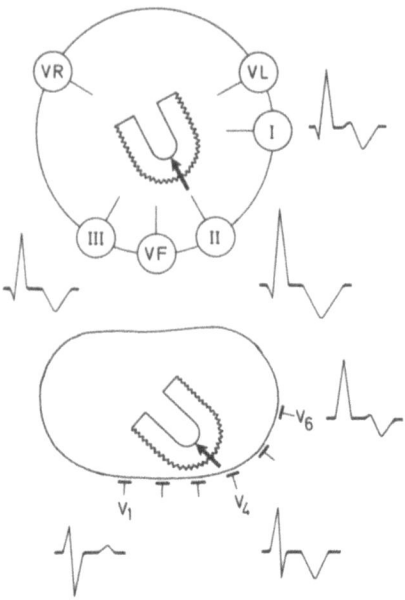

Fig. 59. T vector in ischemia

But apart from delay of repolarization in the outer layers, acceleration of repolarization in the inner layers may theoretically lead to the same result, namely a T vector directed from without inward (Fig. 59). Clinically not unfavorable negative Ts, say due to nervous or metabolic changes or during digitalization, can be explained vectorially in this way.

9.1.4 ECG in Acute Hypoxia ("Asphyxia T")

At times, at the onset of infarction or severe acute coronary insufficiency, a fleeting, very tall positive and widened T is observed in left ventricular leads (Fig. 60). How is this finding explained vectorially? Using again the hypothesis relating to local ischemia, the outwardly directed vector of the positive asphyxial T arises from the slower repolarization of the inner compared with the outer layers, in the subendocardial areas of the heart which, due to the hypoxia, are less well oxygenated. Hence, the outer layers are again electropositive, i.e., repolarized, whereas this process is not yet concluded in the inner layers. Thus, in acute hypoxia of early coronary occlusion, the vector of repolarization is directed outward. An electrode near the epicardium registers a positive T, since the positive tip of the vector points toward it.

70

However, if the outer layers are also poorly vascularized due to the infarction, repolarization is here still more retarded than in the subendocardial areas. The positive asphyxial T changes into the typical T of ischemia with its terminal negativity, as is usually observed in later stages of acute coronary insufficiency and infarction.

9.1.5 ECG in Chronic Coronary Insufficiency (Subendocardial Injury)

Since the inner layers of the myocardium are supplied by the microcirculation of the coronary vessels, a general deficient blood supply of the heart is first noticed in them. This chronic coronary insufficiency causes metabolic disorders, initially of subendocardial muscle cells, which also induce changes in electric conduction.

How does the ST depression come about with changes in the inner layers?

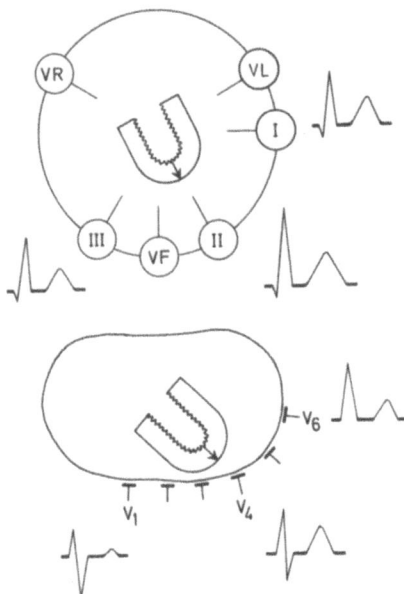

Fig. 60. Asphyxial T

Figure 61 shows a vector that can occur in the ST-T segment at the end of depolarization in coronary insufficiency, i. e., in a period when normally no potential differences ought to exist within the fully depolarized (electronegative) myocardium. It is assumed that the

71

subendocardial layers (hatched in Fig. 61) are less acti
depolarized, and remain electropositive relative to th
Therefore, the ST-T segment will be depressed in the i:
completed depolarization (ventricular complex) anc
repolarization (T wave). For in this interval, the ST ve
from without inward due to the potential difference be
depolarized, i. e., electronegative outer layers, and the l(
i. e., electropositive inner layers. Projection of this vectoi
and also in left precordial leads in the horizontal plane ·
tail end of this vector — will produce negativity, i. e., de
ST-T segment below the zero line.

9.2 Sites of Myocardial Infarction

Since occlusion of large or small branches of the coronar
considered the trigger of cardiac infarction, the locatior
be restricted to regions that are subject to more or less
deficiencies from it (Fig. 62). The loss of myocardium va
on the available collateral circulation.

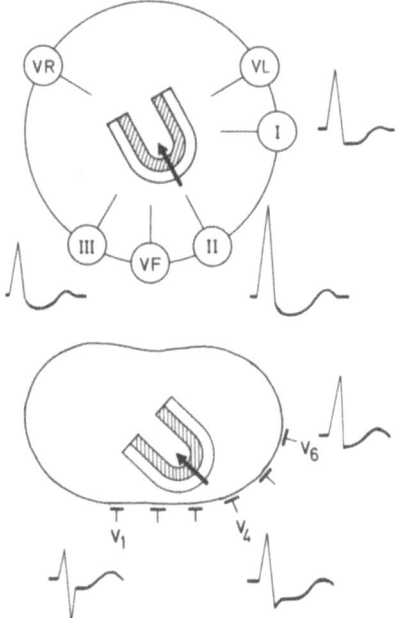

Fig. 61. :
of inner la

72

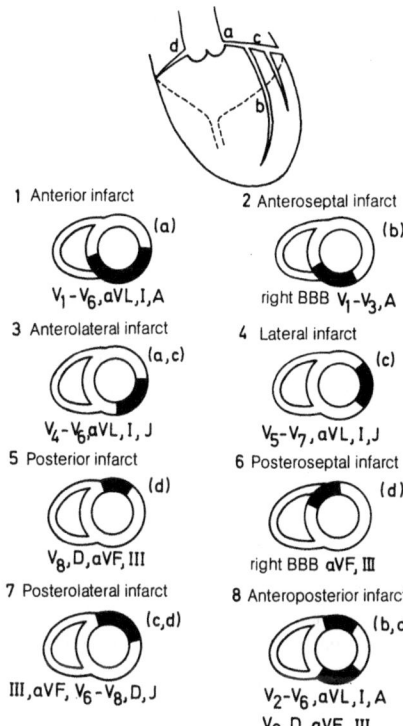

1 Anterior infarct   (a)

V_1-V_6,aVL,I,A

2 Anteroseptal infarct   (b)

right BBB V_1-V_3,A

3 Anterolateral infarct   (a,c)

V_4-V_6,aVL, I, J

4 Lateral infarct   (c)

V_5-V_7, aVL, I, J

5 Posterior infarct   (d)

V_8,D,aVF,III

6 Posteroseptal infarct   (d)

right BBB aVF, III

7 Posterolateral infarct   (c,d)

III,aVF,V_6-V_8,D,J

8 Anteroposterior infarct   (b,d)

V_2-V_6,aVL,I,A
V_8,D,aVF, III

Fig. 62. Site of coronary occlusion and infarcted area

In order to diagnose the site of an infarct, necessary for assessment of *extent* and thus prognosis of the infarction, the topographic anatomy of the coronary vessels should be before one's eyes (Figs. 63 and 64).

Both left and right coronary arteries arise in the aortic sinus of Valsalva. The left coronary runs in the groove between left atrium and left ventricle for about 1 cm before giving off the anterior descending branch in the anterior interventricular groove.

Anatomy of coronary vessels

Together with its branches this supplies the anterior wall of the left ventricle, a portion of the right ventricle, the anterior two-thirds of the septum including the right Tawara bundle, and the anterior fascicle of the left Tawara bundle.

The second branch of the left coronary artery runs as the circumflex branch along the AV groove and supplies the lateral wall of the left heart and the lateral third of the posterior wall.

Occlusion of the anterior descending branch causes extensive anterior wall infarction; occlusion of its right branch, anteroseptal infarction; that of its left branch, anterolateral infarction; and peripheral occlusion of the main trunk, apical infarction. Anterior wall infarcts are frequently associated with bifascicular block patterns.

Occlusion of the circumflex branch causes posterolateral infarction (in 10% also extensive posterior wall infarction).

The right coronary artery courses in the groove between right atrium and right ventricle to the posterior interventricular groove. Its marginal branch supplies the right lateral wall of the heart, its posterior descending branch, both ventricles at the diaphragmatic aspect (posterior and inferior wall).

It also supplies sinus node, AV node, the whole bundle of His, and the posterior fascicle of the left bundle.

Occlusion of the right coronary causes posterior wall infarction. If only lesser terminal branches of the vessel are occluded, a posterobasal infarct is distinguishable. In 10% of subjects the posterior wall of the heart is predominantly supplied by the left coronary artery, so that occlusion of its posterior branch may produce posterior wall infarction.

9.2.1 Extensive Anterior Infarct (Anterior Infarction, Fig. 62/1)

This is a combination of anteroseptal and anterolateral infarction due to occlusion of the anterior descending branch of the left coronary, including all its ramifications. Mainly affected are the anterior wall of the left heart and the anterior two-thirds of the septum; hence, conduction defects are not uncommon with this infarct.

Direct signs of infarction (Q of necrosis, ST elevation of injury, and T of ischemia) are seen, therefore, in almost all chest leads (V2 to V6) and

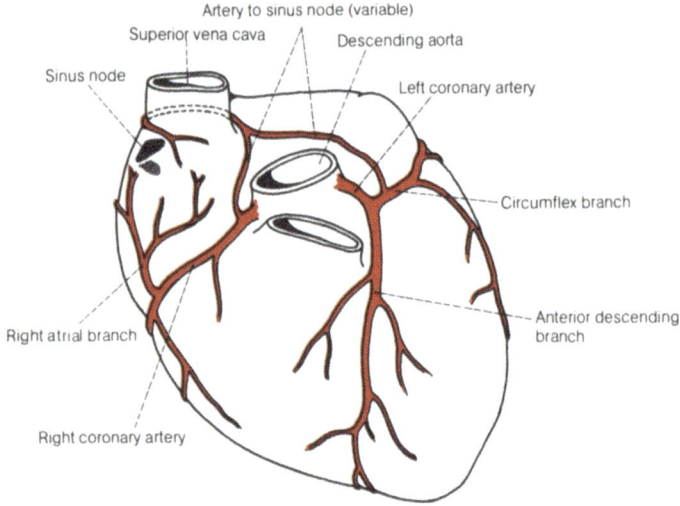

Fig. 63. Topography of coronary vessels. Anterior view

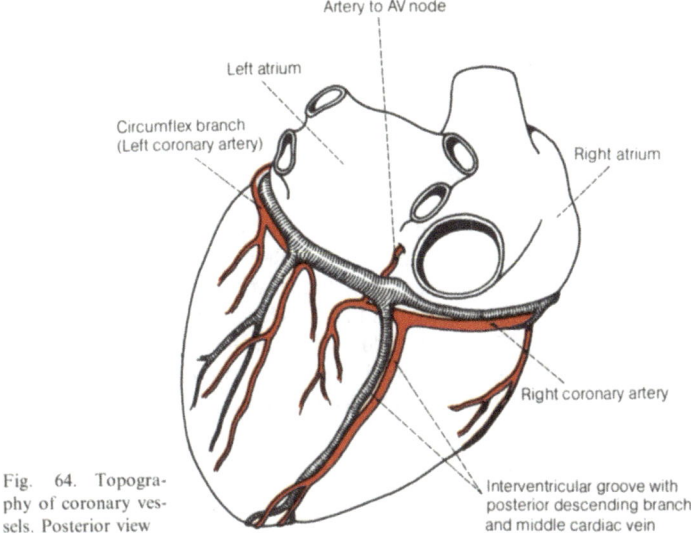

Fig. 64. Topography of coronary vessels. Posterior view

Artery to AV node

Left atrium

Circumflex branch (Left coronary artery)

Right atrium

Right coronary artery

Interventricular groove with posterior descending branch and middle cardiac vein

in the left lateral limb leads I (II) and aVL. The infarcted area lies near these leads. The opposite leads, in this case the subdiaphragmatic leads III and aVF, record only indirect signs of infarction and become mirror images of the direct leads (ST depressions and positive T waves) (Fig. 65).

9.2.2 Anteroseptal Infarct (Infarction of Anterior Septum, Fig. 62/2)

This is caused by occlusion of the right branch of the anterior descending branch of the left coronary. Hence, direct signs of infarction are seen only in leads V1, V2, and V3, whereas indirect signs do not usually appear in other leads. Conduction disorders occur here also due to the affected septum.

9.2.3 Anterolateral Infarct (Anterior Lateral and Anterior Infarction of the Lateral Wall, Fig. 62/3)

This follows occlusion of the left branch of the anterior descending branch of the left coronary. Direct signs of infarction are observed in near leads I (II), aVL, and (V4), V5, and V6. Small infarcts may cause direct signs only in V5 and V6. Indirect signs are possibly seen in V1 and V2.

9.2.4 Lateral Infarct (Fig. 62/4)

This is situated more laterally than anterolateral infarct and affects aVL, I, J, V5–V7.

9.2.5 Posterior Wall Infarct (Posterior Infarction, Fig. 62/5)

Occlusion of the posterior descending branch of the right coronary is the cause in 90% of cases. Direct signs are observed in leads (II), III, and aVF, which are close to the infarct "under the diaphragm". Additional signs may be found in Nehb lead D, which runs along the back behind the heart, and in V7 and V8. Indirect signs are not usually found in chest leads. But indications are found in V1 to V6, more often in V4 to V5. They are more common in limb leads I and aVL.

9.2.6 Posteroseptal Infarct (Fig. 62/6)

In rare cases only small segments of the posterior septum may be infarcted. These are demonstrable only in esophageal and Frank leads.

9.2.7 Posterolateral Infarct (Posterior Lateral Infarction, Fig. 62/7)

This also induces direct signs in leads III and aVF, and additionally in V6 to V7, and Nehb D. Indirect signs may appear in V1, V2, and V3.

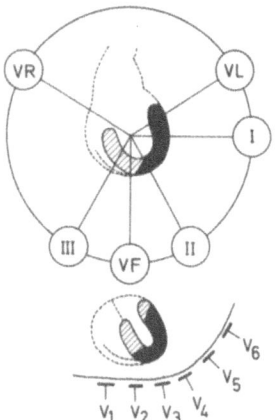

Fig. 65. Diagram of lead projections relative to the topography of anterior wall infarction

9.2.8 Multiple Infarcts (e.g., Anteroposterior Infarction, Fig. 62/8)

A second infarct may intensify the first or remain silent. A massive posterior wall infarct could theoretically "swallow" an anterior wall infarct by its indirect signs, but is not normally capable of doing so, since the precordial leads lie so close to the anterior wall infarct that they register its direct signs rather than the indirect signs of the posterior wall infarction. Therefore, ST depressions in chest leads are due to nearby inner layer infarction rather than to the mirror image of a posterior wall infarct.

9.2.9 Apical Infarct

This arises from occlusion of peripheral portions of the anterior descending branch of the left coronary and frequently provokes direct signs of infarction only in lead V4. In addition, there is low voltage in limb leads. Indirect signs (mirror image) are absent.

9.2.10 Posteroinferior Infarct (Inferior Infarction of Posterior Wall)

Apart from the classic signs of posterior wall infarction in (II), III, and aVF, changes due to infarction are occasionally seen in V1 and VE (exploring electrode over xiphoid process).

9.2.11 High Infarcts

These produce direct signs of infarction only in proximal chest leads and occur mostly laterally. Their extent is commonly small. Corresponding to an anterolateral infarct, direct signs appear in high anterolateral infarction in the 2nd, 3rd, or 4th ICS in V4, V5, and V6, with high posterolateral infarct in V6, V7, and V8.

9.2.12 Subendocardial Infarct (Inner-Layer Infarct)

Directs signs of infarction are ST depressions in all chest leads; if extending laterally, also in I and aVL. T waves may be positive in this case (repolarization changes are against the rule). The ventricular complex itself, i. e., a large part of the myocardium, is not involved electrocardiographically. This infarct can be diagnosed only in the presence of a corresponding clinical picture.

9.3 Course and Classification of Infarcts

The ECG "evolution" of infarction is represented in a mnemotechnic diagram in Fig. 66.

Most frequently a doctor who is called to a patient with recent infarction, will be able to record electrocardiographically the stage of "injury" (outer layer changes or monophasic deformation); example (c) in Fig. 66. Usually at this stage, sings of necrosis (infarct Q) are not yet clear or distinguishable from a positional Q.

Also, ST elevation may still be so discreet as to be overlooked by the beginner. Young doctors on night duty mistake many an initial posterior wall infarction because the zero line of the ECG recorder moves about under unfavorable external conditions and masks an ST elevation in lead III.

Several passing changes appear between the normal ECG example (a) and stage (c), e. g., a stage with a tall positive and broad "asphyxial T" (example b), often lasting for minutes only, or a stage of preinfarction with changing symmetric negative T waves in few leads.

Only later — sometimes days — the typical picture of example (d) in Fig. 66 appears.

The stage exemplified in Fig. 66d with Q, ST elevation and negative T wave persists for weeks, during which the ST segment returns gradually to the zero line (example f). Later, both the Q wave and the ischemic type of T may regress, even disappear.

In approximately 50% of all pathologically proven scars of infarction the ECG has become "silent" and no longer permits diagnosis of an infarct.

The heart of a deceased patient who had typical signs of infarction clinically and electrocardiographically need not always reveal visible changes in every instance. Nevertheless, the diagnosis should be insisted on, for the affected area of muscle had, as it were, "no time" to react morphologically because of the rapid course of the disease. On the other hand, one may see ECG patterns of fairly recent infarction with ST elevation over the infarcted area which do not correspond with recent injury but with a ventricular aneurysm existing for many years.

Rule of thumb for diagnosis of infarction

1. ECG diagnosis of infarction is certain only with typical changes in the QRS complex (initial ventricular deflection) *and* complete depolarization.

2. If ECG findings and clinical picture do not conform, the clinical picture is decisive for the time being. In a severe attack of angina pectoris, suspected to be infarction, ECG changes are frequently delayed.

3. *No* definite pathologic substrate can be correlated with a certain ECG stage of infarction, either morphologically or in time. Hence, it must be emphasized that the division into stages (ischemia, injury,

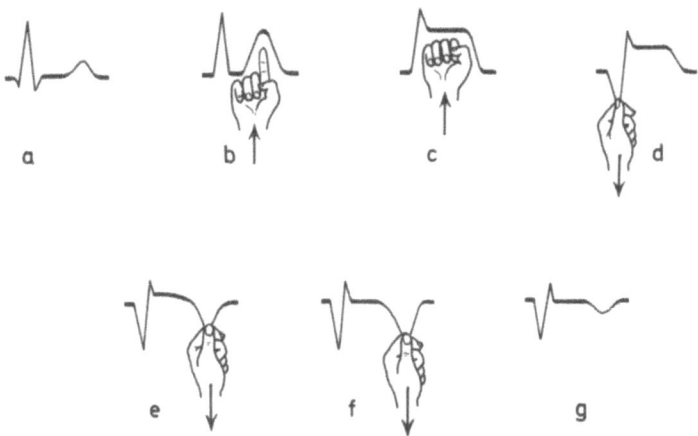

Fig. 66a–g. Mnemotechnic diagram of course and classification of infarction

necrosis, acute, subacute, etc.) is merely an ECG classification and need not correspond with the clinical course (Fig. 67A and B).

9.4 Differential Diagnosis of the ECG in Myocardial Infarction

Should "pitfalls", "doubles", and "masking" of infarct tracings be discussed in a "brief introduction?" Misdiagnosis of infarction has grave psychologic and sociologic consequences for patients: for instance, it is not immaterial whether a patient with the WPW syndrome but a clinically healthy heart is treated for years with anticoagulants because of a supposed posterior wall infarct. To avoid iatrogenic ECG damage, the beginner in ECG ought to be made aware of these problems early on. Besides, vectorial interpretation considerably facilitates differential diagnosis of infarcts.

Differential diagnosis of QRS changes suspected to be due to infarction
   Differential diagnosis between *posterior wall infarct*
   (Fig. 68a–d) and position of Q3
   Acute cor pulmonale
   WPW syndrome
   Extreme left axis deviation
   Differential diagnosis between *anterior wall infarct*
   (Fig. 69a–c) and left ventricular hypertrophy or left bundle branch block
   Chronic cor pulmonale
   Wrong electrode connections (mixing up left and right arm leads)

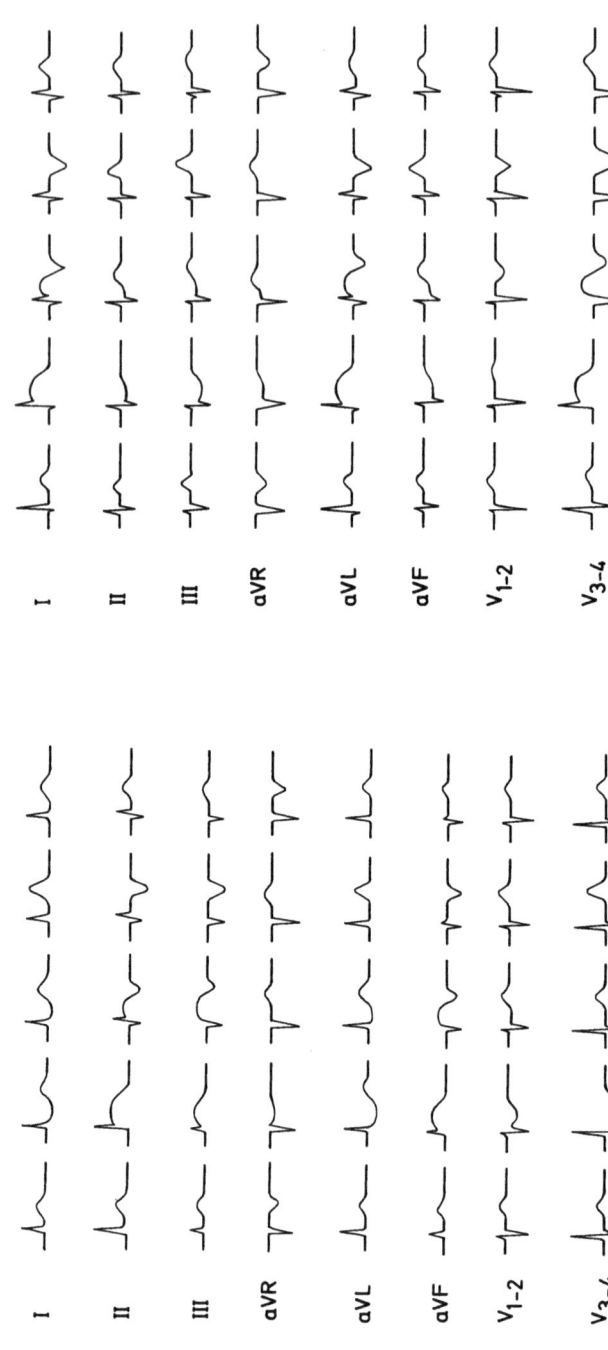

Differential diagnosis of ST elevation suspected to be due to infarction
    Recent pericarditis
    Mirror image of ST depression
    Constitutional ("vagotonia")

Differential diagnosis of (terminal negative) T suspected to be due to infarction
    Outer-layer changes following pericarditis
    Circumscribed "infarct" myocarditis
    Transient ischemic reaction
    Cerebrovascular accident
    Vegetative effects

9.4.1 Differential Diagnosis of QRS Changes Suspected to be Due to Infarction

9.4.1.1 Differential Diagnosis of Posterior Wall Infarct

a) Differential diagnosis between posterior wall infarct and position of Q3. Q3 is observed in raised diaphragm, e. g., horizontal position of the heart in obesity, pregnancy, etc. In these patients, the depth of Q in lead III is clearly changed on deep inspiration. Hence, it is useful to check lead III in deep inspiration and with breath held. Q3 in a posterior wall infarct can become a little smaller on inspiration, but it never disappears completely. When Q in lead III suggests a posterior wall infarct, lead aVF and possibly D in Nehb's triangle and the dorsal chest leads (V7 and V8) must also be recorded. In the presence of a posterior wall infarct there will probably be a broad Q, exceeding 0.04 s, having a depth of more than 25% of the R wave amplitude in one of these leads. But the borders are vague and the diagnosis of posterior wall infarct may be made with a relatively small amplitude of Q3, if the broad Q wave is combined with the typical changes in the ST-T segment which indicate infarction. An additional argument in favor of a posterior wall infarct is a pattern in lead II not resembling lead I, but leads III and aVF (Fig. 68a).

b) Differential diagnosis between posterior wall infarct and acute cor pulmonale. This typical, but relatively infrequent and transitory, ECG pattern is due to acute overloading of the right heart (see Fig. 68b). Among other changes the ensuing dilatation leads to clockwise rotation of the heart on its longitudinal axis (rotation to the left) and hence to a S1 (S2), Q3 pattern. This infarct-suspicious Q3 is not matched by a significant Q in avF. Lead II resembles lead I, whereas it resembles lead III in posterior wall infarct. Usually the diagnosis is arrived at only after serial observations for some time, if ECG tracings are available from the time before or after the event which caused the acute right overload (e.g., pulmonary infarction). The chest leads present a shift of the transitional zone to the left (clockwise rotation of the heart due to the acute dilatation on the right) and the development of ventricular conduction disorders, as (incomplete) right bundle branch block. Occasionally terminal negative T waves are found in V2 and V3 and slight ST elevation due to the ischemia and injury in the overloaded, anteriorly rotated right ventricle. Hence, the terminal deflection does not correspond to the indirect signs of a posterior wall infarct (ST depression and symmetric positive T waves of V1–V3), but could rather be mistaken for a nontransmural anteroseptal infarct (rudimentary supra-apical infarct). P pulmonale is rarely found; this would speak against posterior wall infarction also.

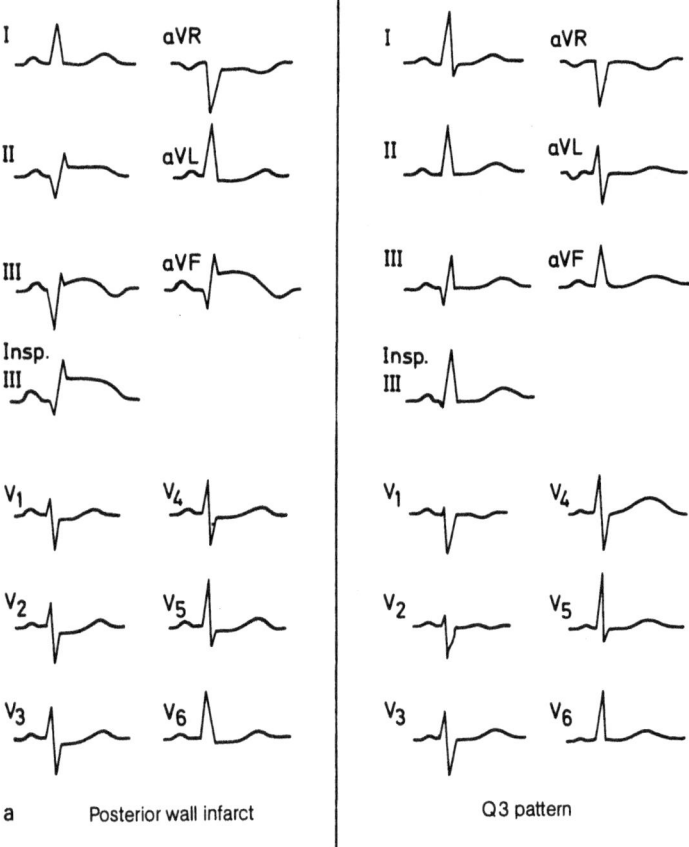

a   Posterior wall infarct   Q3 pattern

Fig. 68a–d. Differential diagnosis of posterior wall infarct

c) Differential diagnosis between posterior wall infarct and WPW syndrome. From Fig. 68c it can be seen that an antesystoly in left axis deviation may imitate a posterior wall infarct. It is not possible to exclude a (former) posterior wall infarct with this type of tracing without knowledge of the patient's history.

d) Differential diagnosis between posterior wall infarct and extreme left axis deviation. A totally negative ventricular complex can also occur in leads III and aVF with marked deviation of the QRS vector to the left and upward posteriorly (in the frontal plane beyond 0°). A summation vector directed more toward aVL causes Q or QS in opposite leads. The precordial leads are essential for clarifying the causes of the abnormal

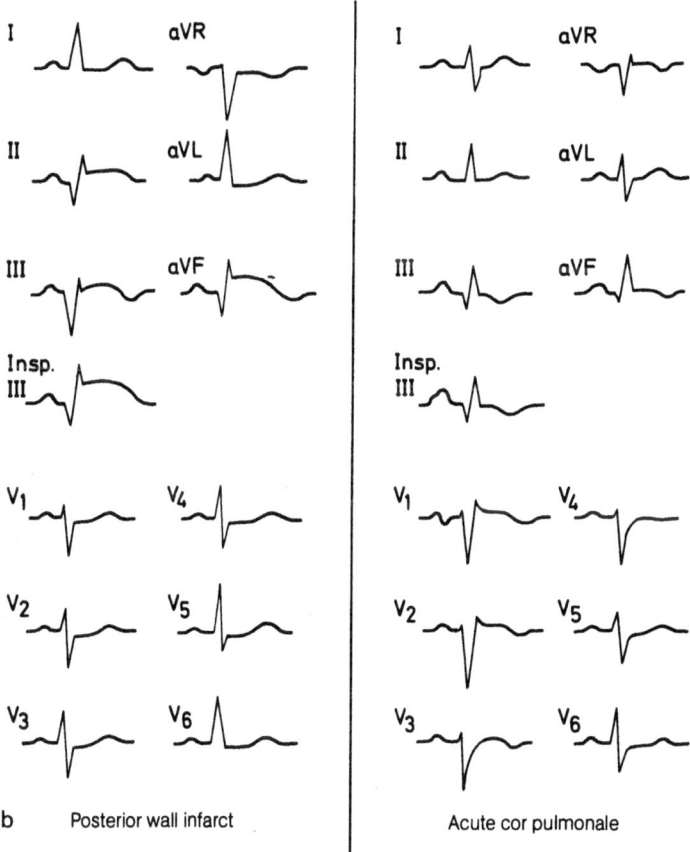

b   Posterior wall infarct   Acute cor pulmonale

Fig. 68. (continued)

axis deviation (extracardiac ones e.g., adhesions; cardial ones e.g., left ventricular hypertrophy or left anterior hemiblock) (Fig. 68d).

9.4.1.2 Differential Diagnosis of Anterior Wall Infarct

a) Differential diagnosis between anterior wall infarct and left ventricular hypertrophy or left bundle branch block. Experience teaches that this is the differentiation which causes difficulties most frequently. Typical of left bundle branch block is the sudden change from QS in the right chest leads to a tall R in left chest leads without a transition zone. In contrast, in anterior wall infarct QS in V2 and V3 is followed by a pattern in V4

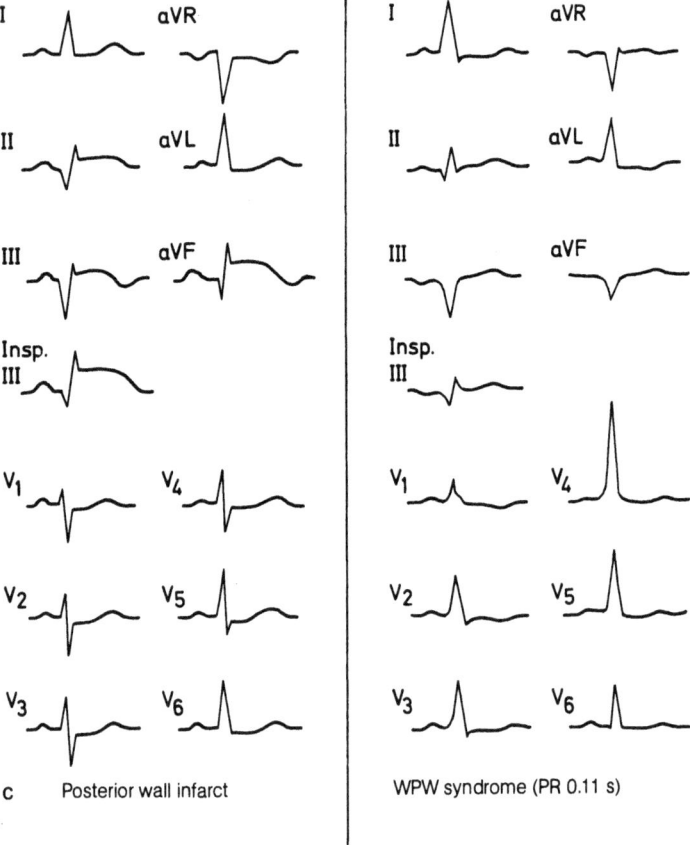

c   Posterior wall infarct   WPW syndrome (PR 0.11 s)

Fig. 68.   (continued)

and V 5 in which the R wave is preceded by a distinct, frequently widened Q wave, which becomes gradually smaller toward V5 and V6 or disappears. Furthermore, any change in the ST-T segment has to be considered in the differentiation. A rule of thumb is that in left ventricular hypertrophy and left bundle branch block the right precordial lead deflections (QRS and ST) are the mirror image of the left precordial ones (Fig. 69a).

b) Differential diagnosis between anterior wall infarct and chronic cor pulmonale. In emphysema there is an rS pattern in all precordial leads due to the low position of the diaphragm and the thus relatively too highly placed normal chest leads (which therefore face the tail of the

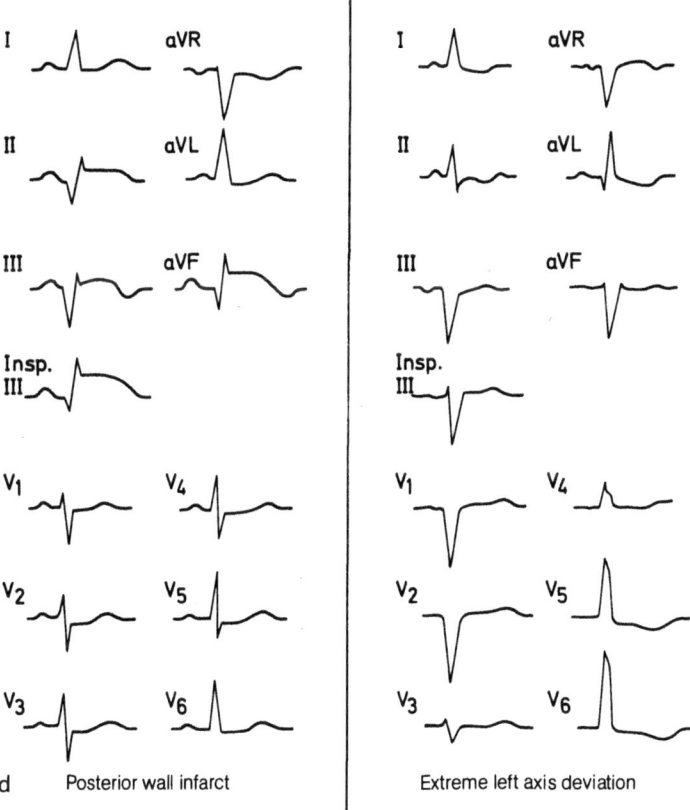

d   Posterior wall infarct   Extreme left axis deviation

Fig. 68. (continued)

85

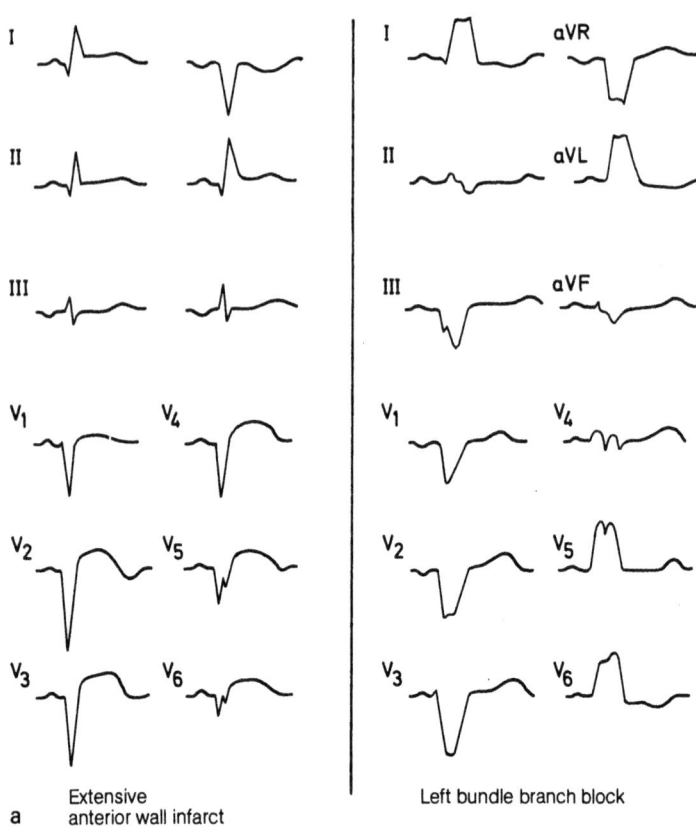

I   II   III

V₁   V₄

V₂   V₅

V₃   V₆

Extensive
a   anterior wall infarct

I   aVR

II   aVL

III   aVF

V₁   V₄

V₂   V₅

V₃   V₆

Left bundle branch block

Fig. 69a–c. Differential diagnosis of anterior wall infarct

summation vector). Occasionally the R waves may be so small that the QRS complex appears to have a QS pattern. Hence, not infrequently septal infarction is wrongly assumed to be present in chronic cor pulmonale. A look at the limb leads helps, however. It reveals deviation of the ventricular axis to the right, and usually a P pulmonale in leads II and III and aVF, as well as typical repolarization changes of right ventricular hypertrophy in leads III and aVF (Fig. 69b).

At times doubtful small r waves can be magnified by application of chest electrodes about a handsbreadth lower near the diaphragm and by recording leads V3r and V4r, in which signs of right ventricular hypertrophy may still be found.

With marked hypertrophy of the right ventricle, e. g., in congenital heart disease, Q is frequently found in V1 and V2 tall R waves.

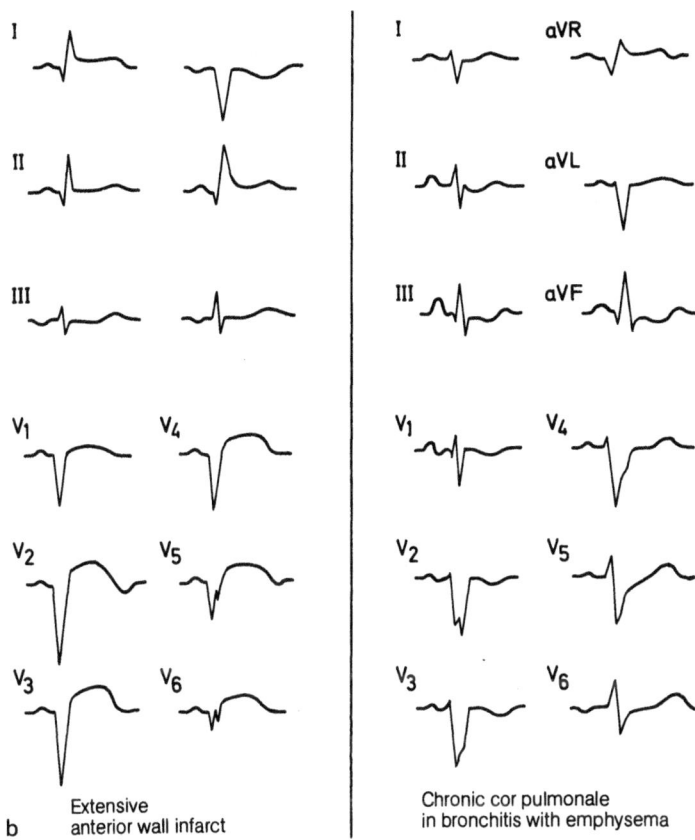

b   Extensive
     anterior wall infarct

Chronic cor pulmonale
in bronchitis with emphysema

Fig. 69.   (continued)

In such extreme right ventricular hypertrophy deep S waves are found in
V 4 and V 5, and rotation of the main vector in the frontal plane above
90° (R in lead III larger than in aVF).

*c) Differential diagnosis between anterior wall infarct and wrong
connections of the arm leads.* When the wires connecting the right and left
arms are exchanged, the initial vector projection on leads I and aVL are
artificially reversed. These leads then register negative ventricular
complexes (QR, rS, QS), which simulate an anteroseptal infarct in limb
leads I and aVL (Fig. 69 c).

Wrong electrode connections are recognized by:
a) Negative waves in leads I and aVL.

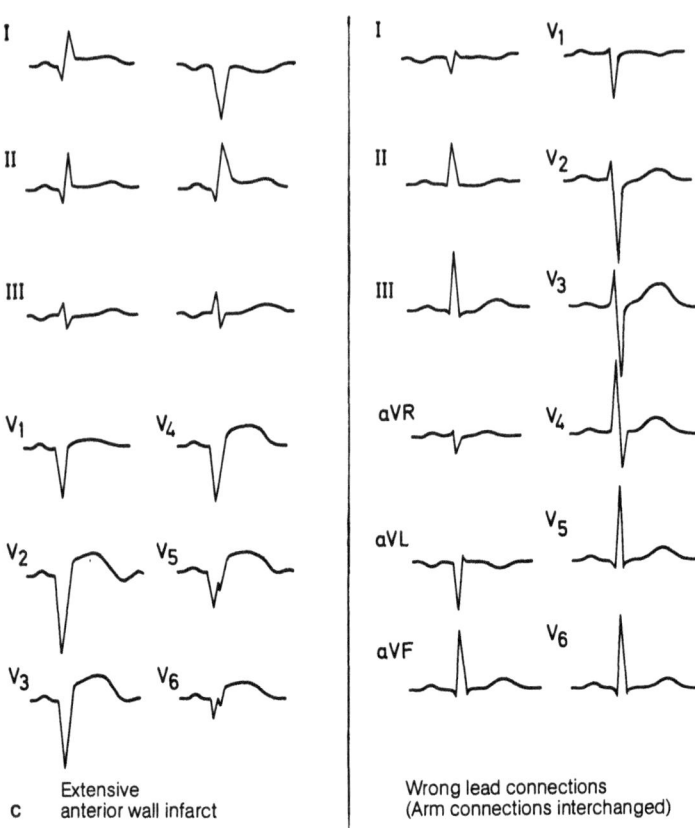

Extensive
anterior wall infarct

c

Wrong lead connections
(Arm connections interchanged)

Fig. 69.   (continued)

b) A positive QRS complex in aVR, where the chest leads V1–V3 do not confirm a right ventricular conduction disorder

c) Absence of an infarct-suggestive Q in leads II and V1 to V6

9.4.2 Differential Diagnosis of Infarct-Suggestive ST Elevation

Elevation of the ST-T segment occurs, apart from recent coronary infarction (outer layer changes), in:

1. Recent pericarditis of different etiologies (provided myocarditis develops near the epicardium).

In distinction from infarction:

a) ST elevation in all leads, especially in II

b) The elevated ST does not directly arise from the descending R limb, but there is an elevated take-off from an S wave — if present;

2. *As mirror image* (indirect signs) opposite those leads with ST depression; e. g., in right precordial leads, upward concave ST elevation with + − diphasic T, as left precordial mirror image of a roller coaster pattern.

3. *In vagotonia or constitutionally,* especially over the right precordium ("garland-like", upward concave elevation).

9.4.3 Differential Diagnosis of Infarct-Suggestive (Terminal Negative) T

A (terminal) negative "coronary" T occurs, apart from ischemia in conjunction with infarction, as a result of:

1. Outer layer changes following pericarditis (e. g., also following pericardiectomy for constrictive pericarditis) in V1 to V6

2. Circumscribed "infarct" myocarditis or other, not coronary arteriosclerotic disorders of repolarization (e. g., leukemic infiltration) in some chest leads

3. Transitory ischemic reactions in acute coronary insufficiency with angina pectoris

4. Cerebrovascular accidents, particularly subarachnoid hemorrhage (negative, broad, fused TU waves; but positive fused TU waves are more common, QU interval lengthened)

5. Increased vagal tone in young persons, recorded in the parasternal leads

"Even if infarction is certain, T is not always completely symmetrically negative; this applies above all to leads aVF and Nehb D in posterior wall infarct. Thus, the appearance of a 'coronary' T by itself is not yet proof *of*, and absence of this change no guarantee *against,* an infarct" (Heinecker, 1965).

9.5 Infarct and Bundle Branch Block

In Section 9.4 bundle branch block tracings were mentioned among the "doubles" that falsely suggest a diagnosis of infarct. Assessment becomes particularly difficult when a patient with a bundle branch block actually develops an infarct in addition, or if in recent infarction which included the septum a bundle branch block pattern supervenes. Both possible sequences have to be considered. Many a time they are distinguishable only by observing the course and checking the ECG frequently, even daily, especially for changes in the ST-T segments.

Diagnosis of an anteroseptal infarct in the presence of a left bundle branch block may be difficult at times, since in both cases a QS wave may be seen over the right precordium to V3 and V4.

This differentiation can be of special clinical importance, since left bundle branch block is increasingly observed among those patients (hypertension and coronary arteriosclerosis) in whom infarction is common.

One is aided by:

1. Observation of repolarization (above all by checking the course) and

2. comparison of the initial ventricular deflection (QS, q or a decreasing R wave)

in the precordial leads.

To 1. The ST shows a monophasic deformation (upward convex ST elevation) over the infarcted area on acute infarction, whereas in left bundle branch block — without infarction or with an old infarct over the right precordium — an upward concave ST elevation — as mirror image of the left precordial roller coaster pattern — is typical.

To 2. In left bundle branch block, the mirror image of QS of the right precordial leads merges without transition into an R or rsR′ pattern.

In the limb leads, a small q wave in front of the widened R of the left bundle branch block also suggests infarction.

It must be mentioned here that a simultaneous, old supra-apical anterior wall infarct, especially if this is an isolated residual finding, remains unrecognizable in same cases of left bundle branch block.

However, since an uncomplicated left bundle branch block in lead III may present a QS pattern, recognition of a simultaneous posterior wall infarct becomes difficult. Whereas lead II rather resembles lead III in posterior wall infarct, it resembles lead I in uncomplicated left bundle branch block. The change in the ST-T segments in leads II, III, and aVF — indicating a typical infarct — is of use only with recent infarction. The chest leads in co-existent posterior wall infarct do not differ essentially from the chest leads in left bundle branch block without posterior wall infarct.

In summary, it can be said that a left bundle branch block is capable of concealing or simulating a posterior or anterior wall infarct. In these cases, the clinical picture decides. If in doubt, daily ECG checks and frequent serum enzyme estimations are of help.

10. Changes in the ST-T Segment

Distinguished are:

1. *Primary* changes — the disorder affects repolarization only.

2. *Secondary* — repolarization is changed because depolarization is already abnormal. In an interventricular conduction disorder with a prolonged QRS complex (in bundle branch block and ventricular extrasystoles), an alternative path of repolarization corresponds to the abnormal path of depolarization.

Therefore, if an abnormal ST-T segment is observed in the tracing at first glance, the second look should take in the main deflection. Differentiation becomes difficult as soon as primary and secondary ST-T changes are combined (e. g., subendocardial injury due to acute coronary insufficiency with left bundle branch block). In practice, only serial observation with frequent checks allows cautions evaluation and differentiation.

Determination of the ventricular gradient for this purpose is too cumbersome in practice.

Below, only the primary ST-T changes are discussed. For practical and didactic reasons, two large groups of causes are differentiated for diagnosis in the first instance:

10.1 Causes of ST-T Changes

Primary ST-T changes due to cardiac abnormality
  Degenerative heart disease (coronary arteriosclerosis)
  Inflammatory heart disease (carditis)
Primary ST-T changes of extracardiac origin
  Autonomic nervous system disorders (orthostasis, vagotonia)
  Electrolyte disorders (potassium, calcium)
  Intoxications:
    Exogenous (carbon monoxide, sedatives, narcotics, nicotine, digitalis)
    Endogenous (thyrotoxicosis, diabetic, uremic or hepatic coma, Addisonian crisis)

10.1.1 Primary ST-T Changes of Cardiac Origin

10.1.1.1 Absolute or Relative Coronary Insufficiency in Degenerative Heart Disease (Coronary Arteriosclerosis or Mechanical Overloading, e. g., Essential Hypertension, Valvar Disease)

Coronary arteriosclerosis
In genuine chronic hypoxemia of the myocardium, e. g., in an elderly arteriosclerotic patient, varied patterns are found — from sagging ST depression (similar to digitalization; but, incidentally, hardly distinguishable if digitalis has been administered, to upward convex ST-T depression with − + diphasic T ("hypertrophy" ST-T), to a minimal, almost shallow ST depression with only moderately flattened T. This latter ST-T change can be prognostically more unfavorable than a deep ST-T dip (Fig. 70).

There is no reliable rule as to the lead in which typical ST-T changes suspicious of hypoxemia can be found in the frontal plane. It always depends on the axis deviation. In an arteriosclerotic patient with marked emphysema the abnormal T vector will be projected most distinctly on leads III and aVF, but in an obese hypertensive patient with a raised diaphragm, in leads I and aVL. However, both patients will reveal the

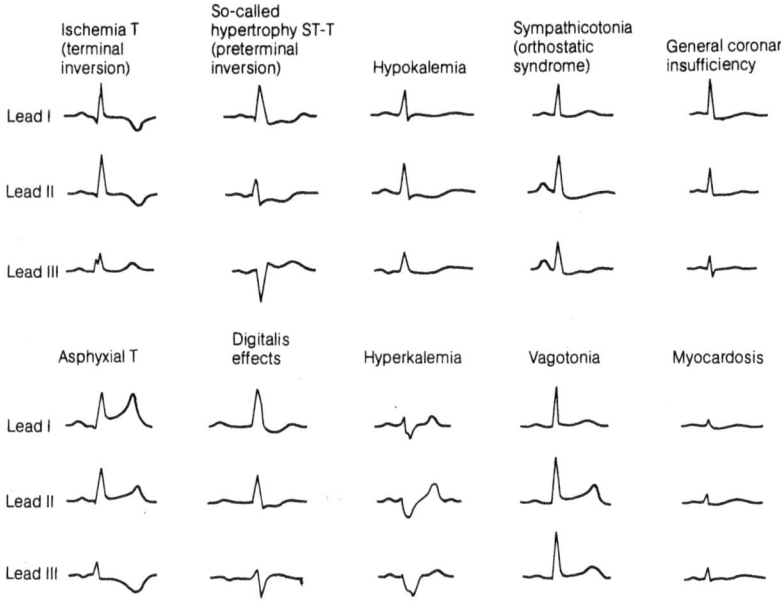

Fig. 70. Differential diagnosis of ST-T changes

ST depression also in V 5 and V 6; this renders e. g., a so-called "right ventricular strain" improbable even in the patient with emphysema.

A conceptual distinction must be made between the rather diffuse "subendocardial injury" of variable etiology with ST depression in many leads, and the more circumscribed "ischemic reaction" (e. g., as precursor and sequel of cardiac infarction) with its symmetric negative T and the barely altered or elevated ST-T segment. It may be mentioned again that in acute hypoxia of the myocardium, a transient, extremely tall positive "asphyxial T" may occur.

10.1.1.2 Inflammatory Heart Disease (Rheumatic Carditis, Viral Myocarditis, etc.)

ECG changes due to degenerative or inflammatory heart disease cannot be distinguished by their pattern alone. Clinical findings and above all, age are of decisive importance. Not every transitory (daily fluctuations!) ST-T depression and T flattening in leads II and III in acute angina or rheumatic fever can be related to myocarditis with certainty. The same picture may arise due to focal toxic disturbance of circulatory regulation in the course of this general disease. Clinical distinction is difficult, but important: not only does it signify the difference between rest in bed for days and weeks, but also the difference between mental stress caused by "myocarditis" in the history and the reassuring knowledge of an abnormal ECG due to harmless autonomic nervous system disturbance. *Carditis*

Different arrhythmias, which are accompanied by a change in ST-T, can be quoted as an argument in favor of myocarditis.

ST-T elevation in all leads occurs only in pericarditis due to inflammation of the myocardium close to the epicardium. This is called subepicardial injury. This finding is more extensive in rheumatic and tuberculous pericarditis than in infarction pericarditis. One finding may be mentioned that must be considered in the differential diagnosis of ST-T elevation, namely the typical ECG of vagotonia, which is associated mainly with low P waves, possibly bowed-upward ST-T elevation, and tall T waves in leads II and III. *Pericarditis*

10.1.2 Primary ST-T Changes of Extracardial Origin

10.1.2.1 Autonomic Nervous System Disorders

Approximately 20%–40% of patients see their doctor about cardiac complaints, but suffer from autonomic nervous system disturbance without demonstrable cardiac damage. It has been mentioned that ST-T changes can be largely similar although they are based on a variety of causes.

Any mental stress is capable of provoking functional changes in the heart via the autonomic nervous system which are hardly distinguishable from those, e. g., of coronary arteriosclerosis without knowledge of the clinical condition.

Proof of mental influence on myocardial function is obtained, e. g., from ECG tracings of patients in hypnosis, when pleasant and unpleasant events are suggested. For instance, the suggestion of an aerial attack caused ECG changes with ST-T depression and flat, even negative, T waves. Psychogenic abnormal impulses were also frequently observed, but conduction disturbance was rare.

Similar changes are registered in the "orthostatic syndrome" after prolonged standing in young patients without evidence of heart disease in their ECG at rest and after exercise or in the clinical picture.

Causes of autonomic nervous system disorders An abnormal ECG, due to autonomic nervous system activity, as recorded most typically in the orthostatic syndrome, requires for its appearance an *enhanced inner readiness:*

Constitutional weakness of connective tissues

Labile endocrine activity (puberty, male and female menopause)

Endocrine disease and hormonal dysregulation (adrenal insufficiency, tetany, thyroid dysfunction),

neurosis or psychosis

Reflexly, due to different organic diseases, especially in the abdomen (cholecystopathy, peptic ulcer, etc.)

Infection and intoxication (abuse of sedatives, nicotine)

Focal diseases (focal infection, neurogenic foci)

and simultaneously *exogenous triggering,* e. g.,

Bioclimatic effects

Unusual physical and mental strain, insomnia,

defective circulatory response after bed rest, uncommon, strong physico-therapeutic stimulation, e. g., sauna baths

The list of causes of primary extracardiac ST-T changes, which is not complete, sets everybody who is to interpret an ECG tracing thinking and makes them cautions from the start.

What distinguishes the "sympathicotonic" ECG?

1. Increase in heart rate
2. Increase in the amplitude of P, which may resemble a P pulmonale
3. Shortening of the PR interval, QRS duration, and also QT interval
4. Flattening of T waves (rarely increase) and "ascending" ST-T depression (Fig. 70).

What is typical of a "vagotonic" ECG?

1. Reduced heart rate
2. Decrease in P amplitude
3. Increase in PR interval, QRS duration, and QT interval (rate dependent)
4. Increased T waves and possibly slight ST-T elevation (Fig. 70).

10.1.2.2 Electrolyte Disturbance

Among electrolyte disorders, only those relating to calcium and potassium are briefly dealt with in Figs. 71 through 73. In the uppermost tracing the normal relationship between first and second heart sound and the end of repolarization is shown. In calcium deficiency, QT is prolonged, which causes the unchanged T wave to terminate after the second heart sound. The degree of the QT prolongation largely parallels the degree of the hypocalcemia.

<small>Calcium deficiency</small>

A hypocalcemic QT prolongation draws attention to the following conditions:
1. Tetany due to absent (postoperative) or inadequate parathyroid glands. In the so-called "tetanoid syndrome" (in hyperventilation tetany), which is usually normocalcemic, there are no corresponding ECG changes.
2. Sprue: practically insoluble calcium soaps in the stools, due to calcium loss.
3. Uremia: Occasionally, the uremic ECG is characterized by a small peaked T wave that follows a prolonged ST-T segment. This special form of T is also an expression of hyperkalemia.

Whereas in hypocalcemia the prolonged QT interval is associated with a T wave of normal duration, in hypokalemia, QT prolongation is simulated because of a wide TU wave. Initially T is flattened, followed by an increasing depression of ST-T, and a positive enlarged U wave, which only appears after the T wave and remains positive (simulated T!) in marked hypokalemia. In the chest leads ST-T may be uncommonly raised and recall infarct patterns. Similar ECG tracings arise in overdigitalization, perhaps due to the frequently concomitant potassium deficiency. But the ECG changes do not always conform with intracellular or extracellular potassium levels; at times they are absent in potassium deficiency.

<small>Potassium deficiency</small>

Since electrolyte disturbance is much discussed in the literature and practice at present, it must be emphasized again that the ECG changes alleged to be typical of potassium deficiency are in fact equivocal. Hence, when potassium deficiency is suspected — as in the treatment of diabetic coma — the ECG changes should not be relied upon.

Figure 71 shows that the QT interval can be shortened in both calcium and potassium excess (a similar picture is found in digitalization). In this case, ST-T is very short, so that the T wave is superimposed directly on the QRS complex.

<small>Hyper-calcemia</small>

This picture may be encountered in parathyroid adenoma and osteitis fibrosa (von Recklinghausen's disease), in widespread metastases of the bone marrow, in myeloma, notably also in bronchial carcinoma without metastasis, in Boeck's sarcoid, and occasionally in hyperthyroidism.

ECG signs of hyperkalemia appear with a serum potassium concentration above 6 mmol/liter (normal: 5.1 mmol/liter, lower limits 4.1 mmol/liter). Initially, tall, spiky, tent-shaped narrow-based T waves

<small>Hyper-kalemia</small>

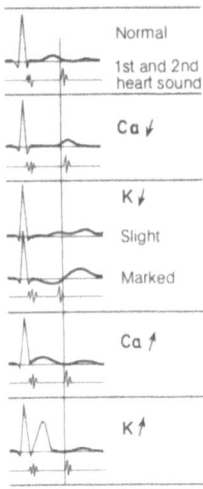

Fig. 71. ECG in abnormal Ca and K metabolism

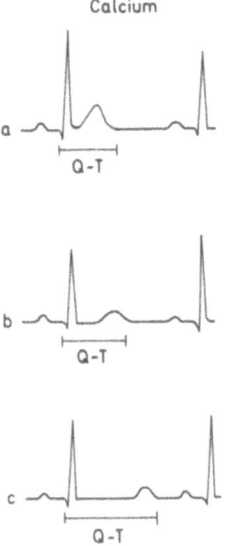

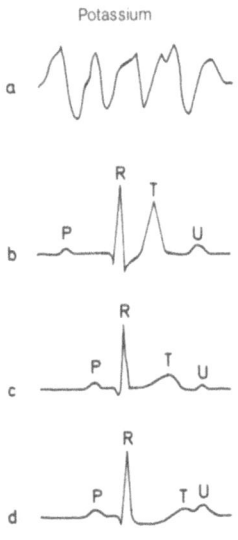

Fig. 72a–c. Calcium. a) Hypercalcemia 8.5 mmol/liter: QT interval shortened b) Normal serum calcium (2.5 mmol/liter): QT interval normal c) Hypocalcemia (1.25 mmol/liter): QT segment prolonged

Fig. 73a–d. Potassium. a) Extreme hyperkalemia (15 mmol/liter): ventricular fibrillation b) Hyperkalemia (9 mmol/liter): prolonged PR interval; tall, peaked T wave; ST segment depressed c) Normal serum potassium (5 mmol/liter): normal d) Hypokalemia (3 mmol/liter): low T wave fused with high U wave appear. The QT interval is basically nonspecific (prolonged in uremia due to simultaneous hypocalcemia). With increasing potassium intoxication the AV interval (PR) is increased (P and R reduced in height, S increased). The ST-T segment is depressed. In addition, conduction disorders appear (intra-atrial, atrioventricular, and intraventricular). QT becomes longer, corresponding with the prolonged QRS, due to delayed and broadened irregular myocardial stimulation. This is followed by atrial fibrillation. After ventricular tachycardia, fibrillation, or flutter, potassium intoxication leads to death.

10.1.2.3 Digitalis

Among the *exogenous toxic effects* on the heart and their subsequent ECG changes the *effect of digitalis* will be discussed because of its particular significance. Again, not all ECG changes are to be regarded as due to intoxication (Fig. 74). Some, especially those under a) and b), ought rather to be evaluated as favorable signs of digitalization. (In order of frequency), the following ECG effects are observed:

a) Changes in ST-T and QT shortening.

b) Enhanced vagus effect on the heart: sinus bradycardia, slowed atrioventricular conduction (prolonged PR interval or even second- and third-degree AV block).

Digitalis signs in the ECG

c) Functional increase in excitability of secondary autonomous centers with tendency to extrasystoles, or ventricular tachycardia and ventricular fibrillation in extreme cases.

To a) Inversion of the T wave and the concave depression of the ST-T segment are explained by accelerated repolarization of the inner layers of the heart muscle. They become electropositive again already during the ST-T segment which causes the T vector to point inward, toward the endocardium, contrary to the normal. In left axis deviation, these changes are encountered in leads I, II, and aVL; in right axis deviation, in leads II, III and aVF.

To b) High digitalis dosage causes sinus bradycardia due to raised vagal tone. This leads to first degree AV block. But digitalis intoxication may also lead to a second-degree AV block similar to a Wenckebach period, or even a third-degree, complete AV block.

To c) In the context of ECG, digitalis can be called the great imitator, as is syphilis among diseases generally. All types of arrhythmias may occur with digitalis. The nearer the foci of excitation lie toward the ventricles, the more is their excitability enhanced by digitalis. Hence, bigeminy of ventricular extrasystoles is frequent. The worst sequel to digitalis intoxication is ventricular flutter or ventricular fibrillation. But higher centers may also be activated, and supraventricular or nodal tachycardia (with AV blockade) can be observed. Winternitz described in 1931 a special digitalis effect on the diseased heart, namely that the

97

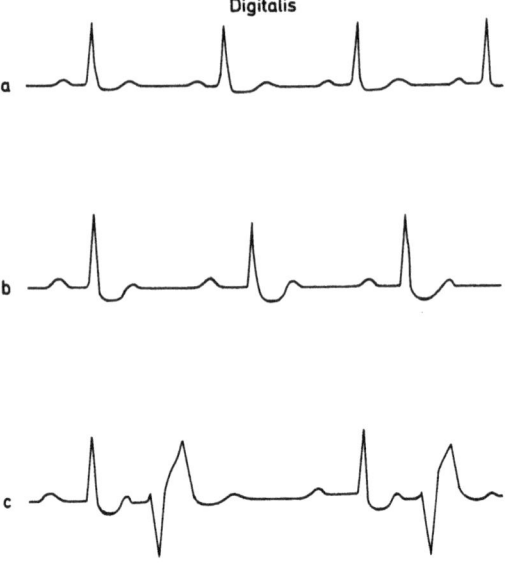

Digitalis

a

b

c

Fig. 74a–c. Digitalis. a) Slight digitalis effect: depression of ST-T segment. b) Marked digitalis effect: depression of J, shortening of QT; slowing of heart rate; prolongation of PR. c) Digitalis intoxication: ventricular extrasystoles, bigeminy. Dangers: total AV block; ventricular tachycardia, ventricular fibrillation.

more diseased and failing side of the heart — usually the left — manifests more marked signs of digitalis intoxication and its abnormal characteristics are enhanced by the drug. The more severely a heart is diseased, the more sensitive to digitalis it is thought to be.

In an emergency, the decision whether a change in ST-T or an arrhythmia is due to too much or too little digitalis (i. e., to the effect of a still inadequate blood supply resulting from cardiac failure) is very difficult to assess. An important argument in favor of digitalis intoxication is the combination of signs from all three of the above-mentioned groups (e. g., trough-shaped ST-T depression, shortened QT interval, PR prolongation, and bigeminy of ventricular extrasystoles).

To conclude this discussion of ST-T changes some remarks are appropriate on how to distinguish "genuine" from "pseudo" ST-T depression and pathologic from nonpathologic exercise response (Fig. 75).

Above all, it should be emphasized that not all ST-T changes in the exercise ECG (e. g., after knee bending until dyspnea occurs) ought to be interpreted as pathologic and the result of coronary insufficiency. The "false positive" exercise test is typified by similar repolarization changes

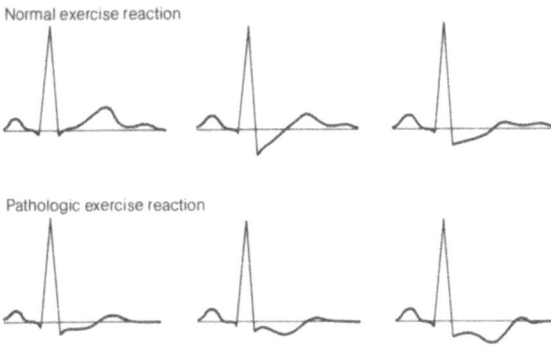

Fig. 75. Changes in ST-T after physical exercise

as the ECG of sympathicotonia and orthostasis: ascending ST depression, (steep rise of ST), flattening of T or even inversion.

10.1.2.4 Simulated ST Depression

In borderline cases it is frequently difficult to distinguish a true ST depression from other varieties. In tachycardia the P wave may fuse with the antecedent T wave: this prevents recording a zero line from which alone ST-T depression can be assessed. The segment between the P wave and the QRS complex can be utilized as "zero line" with reservation only, since depression may also occur in the repolarization segment of the atriogram: at times, this negative wave extends into the ST-T segment, which thus appears to be depressed.

11. Exercise ECG

The effort tolerance test under standard conditions (bicycle ergometer, travelator ergometer, stair climbing according to the method of Kaltenbach and Klepzig), has yielded ECGs that are of prognostic value for the early recognition of coronary disease, especially when compared with the results of angiography. Thus, if in the absence of any abnormal symptoms an effort tolerance test reveals a pathologic ECG, the probability of clinical coronary disease developing within the next 5 years is 85%. In contrast, the risk is only 2.5% in persons with a normal exercise test.

According to present knowledge an effort tolerance test ought to be performed (best by bicycle ergometry) as a prophylactic check-up of the circulatory system when:

1. Symptoms of angina pectoris are reported,
2. More than three risk factors are present in the history (smoking, overweight, lack of exercise, abnormal psychosocial stress) or at examination (hyperlipemia, diabetes, hyperuricemia and hypertension).

Procedure. At the Höhenried Clinic bicycle ergometry has proved best for gradual exercise with the patient sitting on the bicycle. Blood pressure, heart rate, and ECG are recorded at 1-min intervals during a rest period of 3 min, a multistage exercise of 6 (4) min each, and a recovery period of 5 min (dynamometry protocol, see Table 5, p. 104).

Tracings are obtained from leads V 2 (for better recognition of P waves, PR interval, and right bundle branch block), V 5 and V 6. The electrodes are attached to a rubber band and placed around the thorax in the usual localization. To obtain Wilson's central electrode, the electrodes of the limb leads are fixed on the back of the patient, but are not used for registration of limb or Goldberger leads. This method of placing the chest leads, recommended by *Rosenkranz* and *Drews,* has proved to be so good that no advantage is seen in relinquishing it in favor of the disposable electrodes used in intensive care.

Depending on individual capacity dynamometry is usually commenced at 50, 75, or 100 W, but a patient with an infarct is for his first test exercised at only 25, 50, or 75 W during the first 4–5 months after the acute incident. The load is then increased by a further 25, 50, or 75 W after an interval of 6 (4) min each time. As a rule, the exercise tolerance test does not exceed four wattage steps. The patient should always cycle at 50 pedal revolutions per minute.

11.1 Changes in the Exercise ECG Suggestive of Coronary Disease

The behavior of the ST-T segment is the decisive criterion: only demonstration of a horizontal or descending (ischemic) ST depression of at least 0.1 mV in chest leads or 0.05 mV in limb leads and above indicates coronary insufficiency unequivocally. The degree of probability of existing coronary insufficiency, based on the evident ischemic ST depression, is the greater:

Evaluation of the exercise ECG

The more marked these changes

The more leads are involved

The lower the take-off of the ST-T segment

The longer the interval to regression of the ST depression in the recovery phase

The smaller the load during which the changes occur

Causes of a "false positive" exercise ECG
1. Drugs (digitalis, diuretics)
2. Electrolyte disturbance
3. Anemia
4. Valvar disease (aortic stenosis, mitral stenosis)
5. WPW syndrome and other preexcitation syndromes
6. Mitral valve prolapse syndrome
7. Vasoregulatory asthenia and other autonomic nervous system dysfunctions
8. Left ventricular hypertrophy with left-sided injury
9. Block patterns
10. Cardiomyopathies
11. Pericardial disease

Descending or *horizontal ST depression* appearing only on effort or potentiated compared with the ECG at rest is the commonest and most important change in an exercise ECG (see also Fig. 75).

ST elevation is rarely observed, but must be taken seriously prognostically as an expression of subepicardial change. In addition, the following ECG changes occurring during the tolerance test should be considered abnormal:

a) Ectopic pacemakers (supraventricular and ventricular extrasystoles, atrial fibrillation or atrial flutter)

b) Sinoatrial and atrio- and intraventricular blocks

11.2 Doubtful and Prognostically Unreliable Changes in the Exercise ECG

1. An ischemic ST depression in patients digitalized about 10 days prior to the effort tolerance test, must be ignored. *Digitalis* can simulate ischemic ECG changes also in the healthy heart.

101

2. Not all rapidly *ascending ECG changes* are caused by ischemia but by enhanced sympathetic tone, and are of no significance.

3. *Isolated flattening of T* or *T inversion* is likewise mostly due to tachycardia and is not reliable. Changes of negative T waves to positive in the ECG at rest may suggest dyskinesia and early aneurysm in patients after infarction.

11.3 Absolute Contraindications to the Exercise Tolerance Test or Bicycle Dynamometry

1. Recent infarction or suspected infarction
2. Severe angina pectoris
3. Severe arrhythmias, e. g., frequent multifocal or bursts of ventricular extrasystoles at rest
4. Active carditis
5. Any acute infection accompanied by fever

11.4 Relative Contraindications

Relative contraindications to obtaining an exercise ECG (i. e., requiring special supervision by a doctor):
1. Suspected aortic stenosis
2. Atrial fibrillation
3. Implanted artificial pacemakers of fixed rate
4. Conduction disorders with marked bradycardia
5. Any acute infection accompanied by fever

11.5 Criteria for Discontinuation

1. Increasing, severe retrosternal pain, also occurring at other sites, suggestive of angina pectoris, even without preferential typical ECG changes
2. Dyspnea, cyanosis, marked pallor, or general weakness
3. Sudden dizziness as a result of cerebral ischemia
4. ECG changes:
   a) Arrhythmia: frequent multifocal extrasystoles in bursts of three or more extrasystoles, or single extrasystoles falling into the T wave of the preceding cardiac action, paroxysmal supraventricular or ventricular tachycardia, or even atrial fibrillation or flutter.
   b) Disturbance of repolarization: horizontal and descending ST

Table 5. Ergometry protocol.

Patient: Name: ☐☐☐☐☐☐ First name(s): ☐☐☐ Ward: ☐☐☐ Main diagnosis: ☐☐☐

Weight: ☐☐ kg Height: ☐☐ cm Date of dynamometry: 1 9 ☐☐ Dynamometry commenced: ☐☐ o'clock

Circumference of patient's arm: ☐☐ cm Date of birth: 1 9 ☐☐ Room temperature: ☐☐ °C

Digitalis preparation (place cross if "yes") ☐ No. of ergometry during present stay: ☐☐ Humidity of air: ☐☐ %

Rest phase		min	W			W			W			W			Recovery phase		
sRR/dRR	HR		sRR/dRR	HR	Remarks	sRR/dRR	HR	Remarks	sRR/dRR	HR	Remarks	sRR/dRR	HR	Remarks	sRR/dRR	HR	Remarks
		1.															
		2.															
		3.															
		4.															
Complaints		5.															
at rest		6.															

Defining criteria:

objective:

unremarkable course (maximally 4 grades possible) .	(0)
Discontinued because of:	
ECG changes .	(1)
RR behavior .	(2)
HR changes .	(3)
Rise in HR due to fatigue .	(4)
Maximal HR reached .	(5)

☐ ☐

subjective:

No complaints .	(0)
Discontinued because of:	
Pain in heart, pressure in chest .	(1)
Pressure or pain in neck or arm .	(2)
Dyspnea .	(3)
Exhaustion, discomfort in lower limb or joints .	(4)
Headache, vertigo .	(5)

☐ ☐

Cooperation:

reluctant (1)
willing (2)
excellent (3)   ☐

Discontinued, although subjectively, patient could have continued (if "yes": place cross) ☐

_____
(Signature)

103

depression above 0.2 mV in the presence of subjective complaints (in digitalized patients, only marked depression need be considered), monophasic ST elevation.

c) Disturbance of depolarization or severe conduction disorders, e. g., left bundle branch block, second- and third-degree AV block.

With observance of the mentioned contraindications and criteria for discontinuance no death was recorded at the Höhenried Clinic in more than 60,000 bicycle exercise tests in 10 years. Twice, ventricular fibrillation was successfully defibrillated. According to the world literature, a fatal accident during exercise testing can be expected in 1 in 10,000 cases.

12. ECG Diagnosis of Arrhythmias

The diagnosis of disordered rhythms is the specific domain of ECG. However, systematic discussion of all arrhythmias would exceed the purpose of an introductory text.

What is the systematic procedure for correct assessment of a disordered rhythm in the ECG?

Systematic procedure for assessing arrhytmias

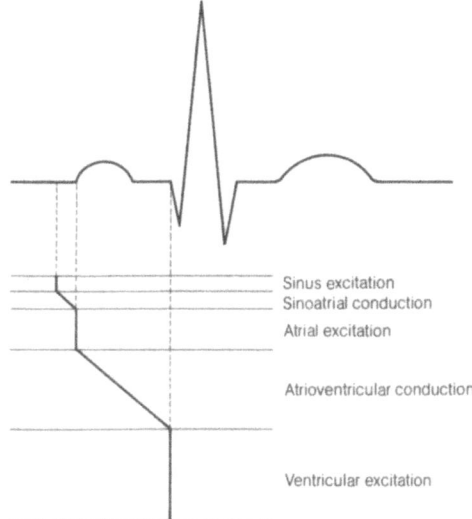

Fig. 76. Diagram of a normal cardiac depolarization sequence as aid to the presentation of the time sequence of impulse conduction

Analysis of complex arrhythmias is easiest when a long strip at a paper velocity of 25 mm s^{-1} is available from that lead which has the clearest definition of the smallest potential changes, namely the P waves. Frequently dividers will be required, since this enables measurement of time relations of certain waves to each other as well as to other segments of the tracing. In some cases establishing an AV diagram (Fig. 76) is useful, particularly for didactic purposes.

105

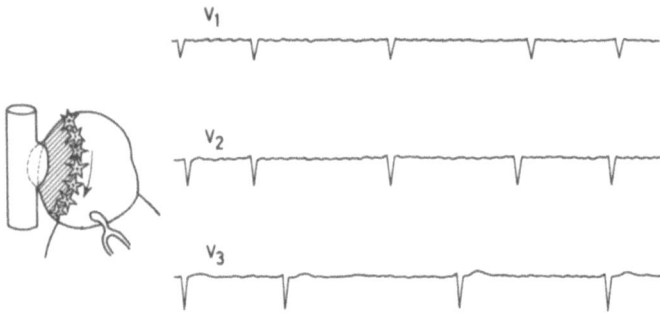

Fig. 77. Atrial fibrillation. The fibrillation waves are best recognized in right chest leads. In the diagram the question is left open of whether the atrial fibrillation is due to "circuit movement" or to "multifocal extrasystoles"

12.1 Are (Normal) P Waves Present?

Atrial fibrillation
Atrial fibrillation (Fig. 77) is one of the commonest arrhythmias. It is characterized by the absence of P waves, appearance of atrial fibrillation waves (f waves) at a frequency of 350–600 per minute, and totally irregular sequence of beats of the ventricular complexes (absolute arrhythmia). The latter have a supraventricular configuration provided there is no co-existent bundle branch block or ventricular aberration due to depressed conduction. Atrial fibrillation followed by regular ventricular activity points to AV block with AV rhythm or ventricular automaticity (Fig. 78). The following criteria indicate aberrant spread of activation during atrial fibrillation (rather than extrasystoles): rsR' in V1, absence of fixed coupling and a compensatory pause.

Atrial flutter
Whereas the waves of fibrillation display a constant change in height and width, the waves of *atrial flutter* appear as regular undulations (F waves) — also called sawtooth waves — (Fig. 79), with a frequency of 220–350 per minute. These, as well as normal P waves and waves of fibrillation, are best recognized in leads II, III, aVF, V1, and V2.

The flutter waves are about twice as high as those of fibrillation but considerably broader, since they include atrial repolarization (Ta). Mixed forms are called flutter fibrillation (impure flutter). Although atrial flutter is relatively rare, its precise ECG diagnosis is eminently important, since treatment is required in every case. In untreated atrial flutter the conduction ratio from atrium to ventricle is frequently 2:1 (Fig. 80a), which results in a ventricular frequency of 120–150 per minute; this is poorly tolerated, particularly by elderly patients. In the presence of this ratio, the atrial flutter in the ECG is often mistaken for a different form of atrial tachycardia and treated wrongly. The rare transition to 1:1 conduction would signify ventricular flutter.

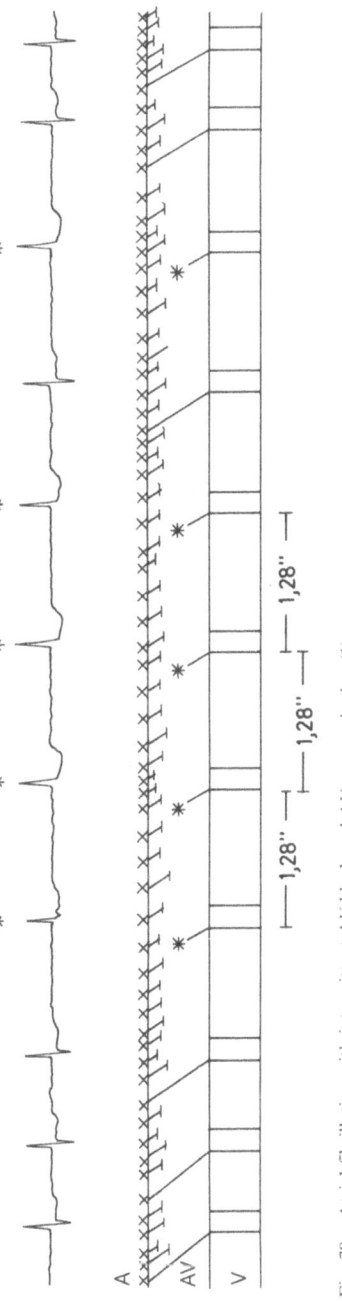

Fig. 78. Atrial fibrillation with intermittent AV block and AV escape rhythm (*)

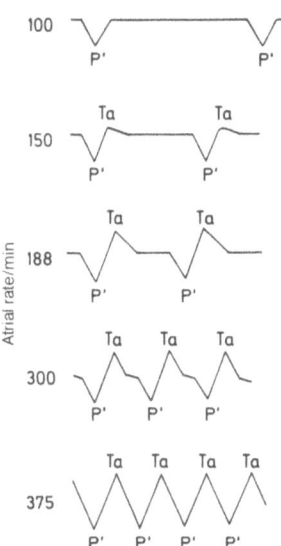

Fig. 79. Rising heart rate from atrial tachycardia to atrial flutter with increasing prominence of atrial repolarization (Ta wave). It is typical of the sawtooth appearance of the atrial flutter waves

107

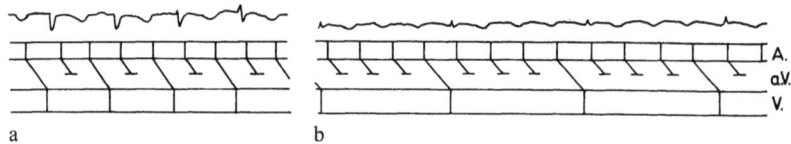

Fig. 80a and b.   Atrial flutter alternating between a) 2:1 and b) 4:1

12.2 What is the Distance Between Individual P Waves?

A sinus frequency below 60 per minute is called sinus bradycardia, above 100 per minute, sinus tachycardia. In marked tachycardia the axis of P ("pseudo P pulmonale") and QRS becomes more vertical.

If the P intervals are measured with dividers (needed again and again for assessing arrhythmias in the ECG), they are very rarely identical. *Sinus arrhythmia,* especially respiratory arrhythmia, is the most common arrhythmia. In young people, the rate is usually increased at inspiration and slowed at expiration. But sinus arrhythmia also occurs independent of respiration in the presence of autonomic nervous system dysfunction, e. g., during recovery from infectious diseases. However, the older the patient, the less should this arrhythmia be considered as normal and physiologic.

Sick sinus syndrome   In the elderly, on the other hand, the *sick sinus syndrome* is often observed. This chronic progressive disease manifests itself most frequently as permanent sinus bradycardia, less frequently as bradycardia alternating with tachycardia: the slow phases are often due to sinoatrial block, the tachycardia due to atrial fibrillation or flutter. The basic disturbance is a morphologic, not a functional defect. The changeable ECG patterns are best registered with an ECG tape-recorder.

Sinoatrial block   In first-degree *sinoatrial block* impulse conduction between sinus node and atrium is prolonged. This is not measurable on the ECG because sinus node activation is not recorded in the tracing. In second-degree sinoatrial block (type I, Wenckebach period), the PP interval decreases progressively till an atrial and ventricular complex lapses (Fig. 81). The discrepancy between a gradual increase of sinoatrial conduction and decrease of PP intervals is only apparent. The analogous phenomenon of the atrioventricular Wenckebach block is easier to understand and will be explained there. In type II an atrioventricular complex is dropped without progressive PP shortening. The pause amounts to double or a multiple of a normal PP interval. The block is constant at 3:2, 5:4, or alternating. A 2:1 sinoatrial block mimics sinus bradycardia. A sinoatrial block may resemble sinus arrhythmia or be present simultaneously.

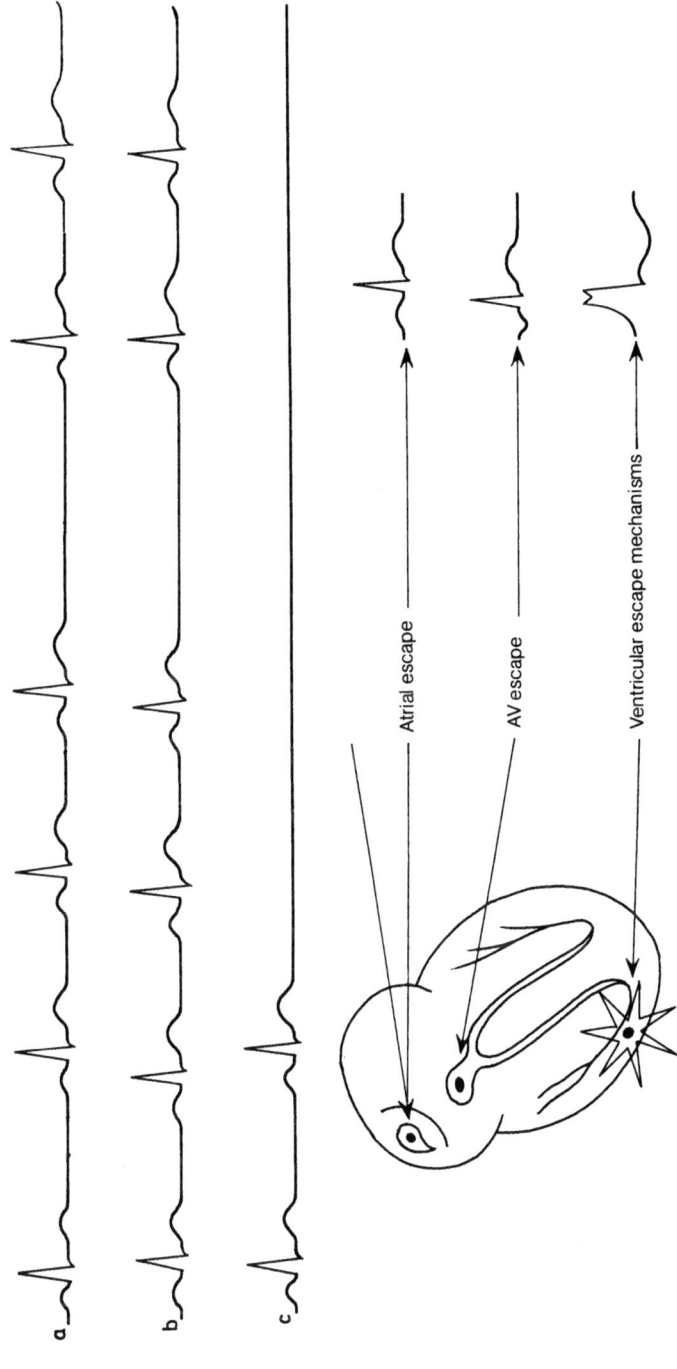

Fig. 81a–c. Sinoatrial block. a) Second degree, type I. Wenckebach period: decreasing PP intervals until dropped beat (P wave and QRS complex). b) Second degree, type II, dropped beat without previous decrease of PP intervals. c) Complete SA block. No escape mechanism has become effective as yet in this strip. Three possible escape centers have been drawn in the diagram

a

b

c

Atrial escape

AV escape

Ventricular escape mechanisms

12.3 What is the Shape of the P Waves?

Distinct lengthening of P in all leads points to an intra-atrial conduction defect. Analysis of the vector position of the atrial stimulation can indicate an abnormal origin of excitation in the atrium or an aberrant Wandering pacemaker spread of the stimulus in this portion of the heart. With a *wandering pacemaker,* the origin of the stimulus is shifted to caudal portions of the sinus node or to more distal atrial segments. Thus, P becomes negative in leads II and III and the PR interval shorter, usually below 0.12 s, whereas the PP intervals are lengthened. Return to the sinus node is by stages or jumps and causes a change in the shape of the P waves from one atrial stimulation to the next (Fig. 82). This type of arrhythmia is common in children and adolescents and is harmless (see Chap. 14).

12.4 What is the Distance of P waves from the Following QRS Complex?

A V block This refers to *A V blocks* of different degree (Fig. 83). In *first-degree A V block* (AV conduction delay), the PR duration (AV interval) is identical for each heart beat, but exceeds the normal PR time of 0.2 s. Two types of *second-degree A V block* are known. Type I (Wenckebach period, Mobitz block I) is characterized by progressive lengthening of the PR

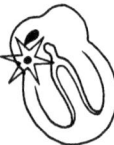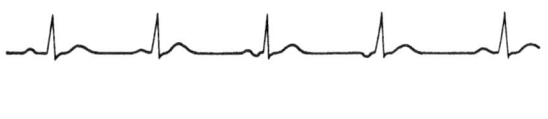

Fig. 82. Wandering pacemaker. The origin of an impulse has been marked in the distal right atrium of the diagram. This corresponds to the position of the pacemaker at the instant of the fourth beat in the respective ECG strip. (Where not specially noted, lead 1 is presented in the diagrams)

interval up to the lapse of a ventricular complex. Since the augmentation in PR interval *lessens* from beat to beat while the PR interval increases progressively, there is a *decrease* in the RR interval (Fig. 83 b). Type II second-degree AV block (Mobitz II) reveals sudden losses of individual ventricular activation at regular or irregular intervals. A 2:1 AV block is one where only every second atrial excitation is conducted to the ventricles. In *third-degree A V block* (complete AV block) (Fig. 84), conduction is completely interrupted in the AV node, the bundle of His, or both bundle branches (Tawara bundles). Atria and ventricles beat

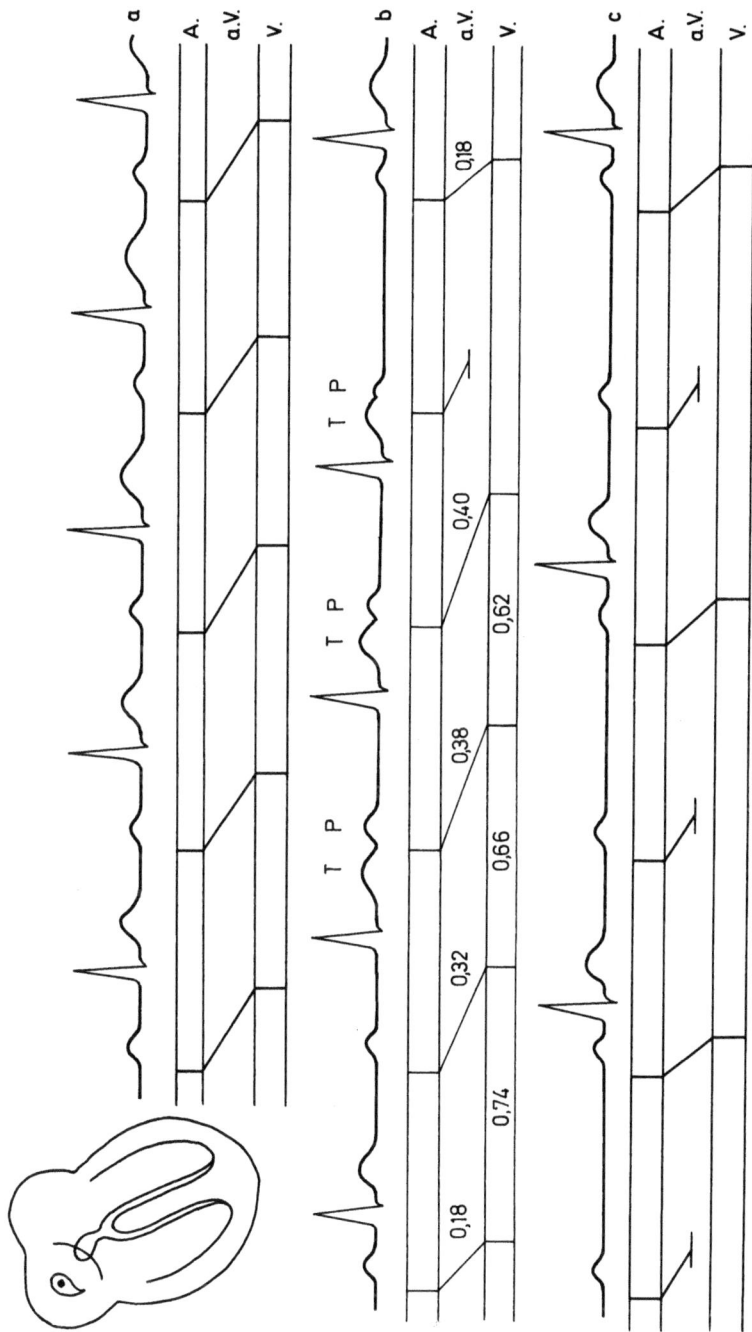

Fig. 83a–c. AV blocks of different degree. a) First-degree AV block. Prolonged AV interval (PR interval). b) Second-degree AV block, type I (Wenckebach period). Subsequent to the 2nd to 4th P wave, the PR interval increase becomes progressively smaller (0.32–0.38–0.40); the RR intervals are thus progressively shortened (0.74–0.66–0.62). c) Second-degree AV block, type II (2:1 block)

111

idiorhythmically (independent of each other) (block dissociation). According to the site of the block, the ventricles respond to a secondary center in the bundle of His distal to the interruption or a still more distal, tertiary center.

The ECG does not reveal with certainty where a first-, second-, or third-degree block is localized. Proximal AV blocks are mostly associated with unaltered ventricular complexes, while distal blocks, particularly of second and third degree, have deformed ventricular complexes, as seen in bundle branch block. But these signs are unreliable, since a proximal block may be present in addition to a distal conduction defect in a Tawara bundle. This can be clarified only by means of a His electrogram.

His bundle electrogram   Figure 85 shows the relations between ECG and His electrogram. The latter, obtained with a catheter electrode introduced via the right femoral vein across the tricuspid valve, records directly from the conduction system. It permits subdividing the AV interval, normally ranging from 0.12 to 0.19 s, into an AH interval (atrium to His interval:

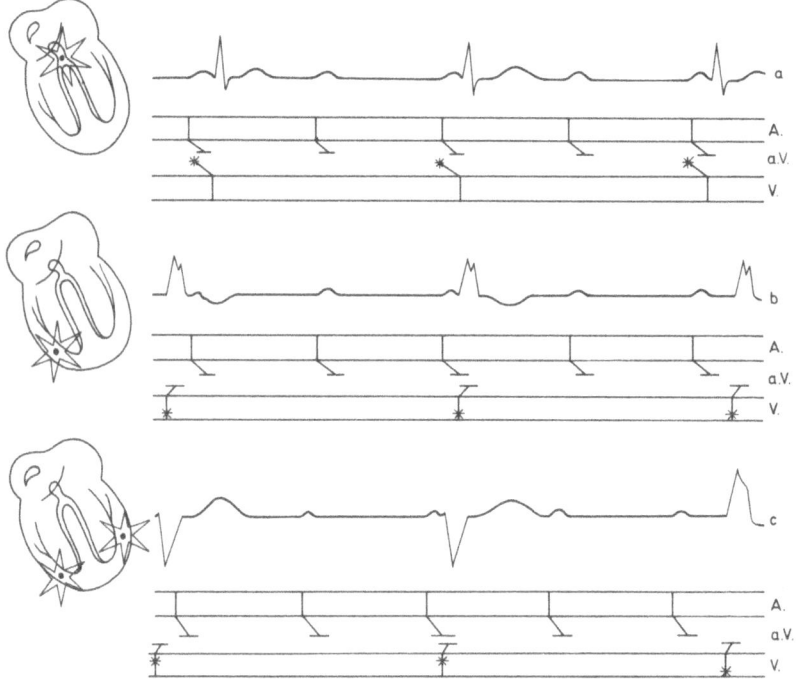

Fig. 84a–c.   Third-degree AV block. a) With AV escape rhythm. b) With idioventricular rhythm, originating in the right ventricle. c) With two different escape rhythm centers in the right or left ventricle

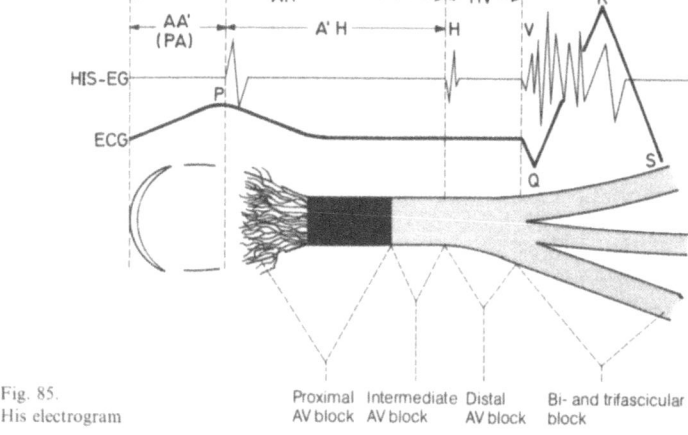

Fig. 85.
His electrogram

Proximal Intermediate Distal   Bi- and trifascicular
AV block AV block   AV block   block

0.08–0.14 s), and an HV interval (His to ventricle interval: 0.03–0.05 s). If the action potentials of neighboring segments of the right atrium are registered at the same time, the AH interval can be further divided into an AA′ (PA) interval of 0.025–0.045 s and an A′H interval of 0.055–0.12 s. The former corresponds to depolarization within the right atrium, the latter to that in the AV node. The H wave corresponds to the electric stimulation of the bundle of His. AV blocks can be located proximal or distal to it.

Prognosis is better in proximal than in distal AV blocks, since in the former the bundle of His may substitute as secondary center for generation of impulses with a rate which can still be influenced by the autonomic nervous system. As mentioned in Table 1 (p. 48), the PH or AH interval is prolonged in first-degree proximal AV block: it is the time from atrial stimulation to activation of the bundle of His. The HV interval remains unchanged. In a second-degree proximal AV block, a Wenckebach period is almost always present. This is characterized in the His electrogram by an increasing lengthening of the PH interval and a constant HV interval with occasional dropped beats as a consequence of interrupted conduction (Mobitz type I). Proximal
AV block

Third-degree proximal AV block leads to complete interruption of the bundle of His near the AV node. In this case, the impulses are initiated in the preserved distal portions of the bundle of His. The heart rate is usually between 40–50 beats per minute. If no additional bundle branch block is present, ventricular complexes are not deformed and not widened.

In distal AV block, generation of impulses travels undisturbed from the sinus node via atria, AV node and bundle of His to the H wave. The Distal
AV block

113

delay or interruption lies distal to it. This may either be a block or conduction delay in the distal bundle of His or in the Tawara fascicles. Here also one distinguishes first-, second-, or third-degree AV block. The first-degree distal AV block is usually due to retarded conduction in all three Tawara divisions. The second-degree distal AV block shows no Wenckebach period, but intermittent absence of ventricular complexes (Mobitz II) — while conduction time between atria and ventricles remains constant, so that there are more P waves than QRS complexes. As mentioned, the block can occur at a regular sequence of 2:1, 3:1, or 4:1. In the His electrogram, the PH or AH interval is normal, whereas the HV interval is prolonged or interrupted. The further distal the disorder in the bundle of His, the closer it approaches the branching of the Tawara divisions. Frequently both the left anterior fascicle and the right fascicle are blocked, rarely the left posterior fascicle. In this manner, bi- and tri-fascicular blocks originate. The last correspond to a total AV block and require a ventricular escape rhythm whose QRS complex is deformed like a right bundle branch block if situated in the left ventricle, and like a left bundle branch block, if in the right ventricle. Its rate is around 20–30 beats per minute.

AV block in atrial fibrillation In 20% of all AV blocks atrial depolarization is not controlled by the sinus node but there is atrial fibrillation (cf. Fig. 78) or flutter, an ectopic atrial rhythm or atrial extrasystoles. Under these conditions the diagnosis of an AV block is obviously much more difficult and can only be assumed if there are strictly uniform QRS intervals (due to the AV escape rhythm).

12.5 What is the Distance Between Apparently Identical Ventricular Complexes?

12.6 What is the Time Relation of Differently Shaped Ventricular Complexes to Each Other or to the Basic Rhythm?

These two questions are connected and have to be asked wherever ventricular complexes of different pattern appear. Once it has been ascertained that dissimilar ventricular complexes are not due to transitory intraventricular conduction delay, the anomalous QRS configuration must be ascribed to a *ventricular heterotopic or ectopic pacemaker*. Widening and deformation result from a retarded and vectorially deviating spread of ectopic potentials, which are not conducted via the conduction system but via the contracting myocardium (nonpreferential pathways). Enhanced automatism of subordinate centers may have many causes: psychologic influences, release of

114

catecholamines, local hypoxia, hypercapnia, pH changes, distention of myocardium, change in calcium or potassium concentration, drugs such as digitalis, etc. When there are ventricular complexes of varying morphology, the basic rhythm must be distinguished from:

Extrasystoles
Escape systoles
Escape rhythms
Parasystoles (para-arrhythmia)

12.6.1 Extrasystoles

Extrasystoles are premature contractions of the heart or of a segment of the heart. If the interval from the previous normal beat is constant it is called fixed coupling. Extrasystoles are the commonest disorders of impulse generation.

The following are distinguished:

1. *According to the site of origin:* supraventricular and ventricular extrasystoles. In the case of atrial extrasystoles and AV extrasystoles the ventricular complexes generally have the same shape as the ventricular complexes of the basic sinus rhythm, since the excitation is conducted in a similar fashion via the AV node. However, due to aberrant conduction they can at times display appreciable changes of ventricular complexes, mostly like a right bundle branch block. Exact localization of the focus of supraventricular extrasystoles is feasible by careful scanning of the P waves (Fig. 86). Sinus extrasystoles produce P waves that are identical with those of the basic rhythm, whereas so-called atrial extrasystoles have divergent P forms. Since according to recent studies, the AV node does not contain any pacemaker cells, those ectopic beats hitherto called AV extrasystoles, should be called His extrasystoles. But the conventional terminology will be retained here.

Either no P wave precedes the AV extrasystoles (as in the "middle nodal rhythm"), or the atrium which is depolarized simultaneously with the ventricles from the AV node registers a negative P wave preceding the ventricular complex by an interval of 0.12 s (as with the "upper nodal rhythm"), or immediately follows the QRS (as with the "lower nodal rhythm") (cf. Fig. 88d, p. 119). Coronary sinus extrasystoles, observed during cardiac catheterization, also have a negative P wave which, however, precedes ventricular depolarization by more than 0.12 s.

Occasionally, when supraventricular extrasystoles occur early, the P wave is superimposed on the preceding T wave, which masks the atrial wave (TP grafting).

Blocked supraventricular extrasystoles consist of P waves that are not followed by a ventricular complex because the conduction system is still in a refractory state.

Supraventricular extrasystoles

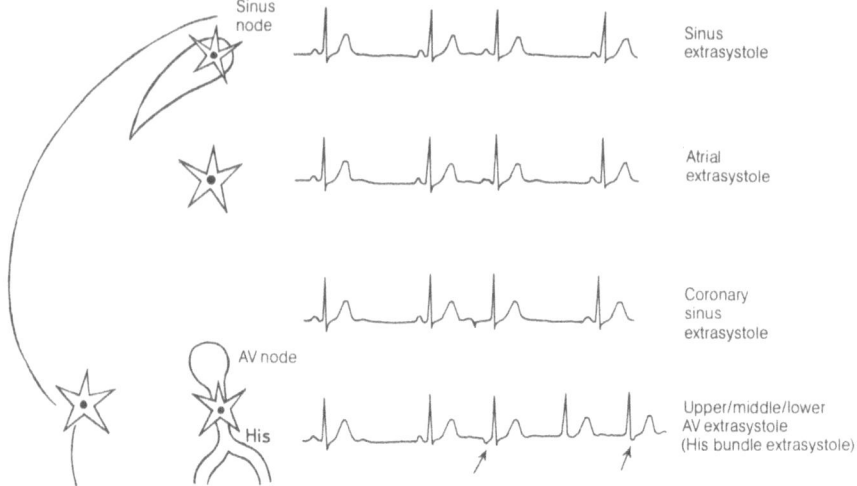

Fig. 86.   Supraventricular extrasystoles

Ventricular extrasystoles   In ventricular extrasystoles the stimulus originates in the ordinary ventricular myocardium. The pattern resembles a bundle branch block the more the further the site of origin is from the A-V node. While it is true that septal extrasystoles are somewhat widened, they still resemble that seen with the basic rhythm. Right ventricular extrasystoles present a ventricular complex resembling a left bundle branch block, left ventricular extrasystoles resembling a right bundle branch block (Fig. 87). Ventricular extrasystoles mostly follow the preceding normal beat at a fixed coupling interval. If this is not so (gliding coupling), the existence of parasystole must be borne in mind, or the extrasystoles are of multifocal origin.

Combined systoles   Fusion of a ventricular extrasystole with a nomotopic ventricular depolarization yields a combined systole (fusion beat), which presents a mixture of characteristics of the normal and the extrasystolic ventricular tracing.

2. *According to the morphology:* monomorphic unifocal and polymorphic multifocal extrasystoles. Multifocal extrasystoles, i. e., those of variable shape, are prognostically less favorable than unifocal ones.

3. *According to incidence:* occasional — frequent (e. g., bigeminy, when each normal beat is followed by an extrasystole) —bursts (or runs) of extrasystoles.

R on T phenomenon   In organic cardiopathies, especially in infarction, the so-called R on T phenomenon is clinically significant, because dangerous ventricular arrhythmias can be expected. These are very early ventricular extrasystoles the QRS complex of which closely approaches the vulnerable phase of the previous normal or ectopic excitation, i. e., at or just before the T peak (see also Fig. 87c).

4. *According to its response to the basic rhythm: compensated* extrasystoles. In these, the refractory period of the extrasystolically activated ventricle has not yet ended, which causes the subsequent normal (sinus) stimulation not to be conducted. This gap is called "compensatory pause." Hence, compensated extrasystoles the sum of two normal RR intervals, measured from the first to the third R, is equal to the sum of the RR intervals before and after the extrasystole. (Fig. 87c). The sinus rhythm is prematurely interrupted by atrial extrasystoles, AV extrasystoles, or rarely, by retrograde conduction of the ventricular extrasystole to the atria; but resumes at the initial rhythm. Contrary to most ventricular extrasystoles, the postextrasystolic pause is incompletely compensated, i. e., it is shorter than twice the normal RR interval.

Compensatory pause

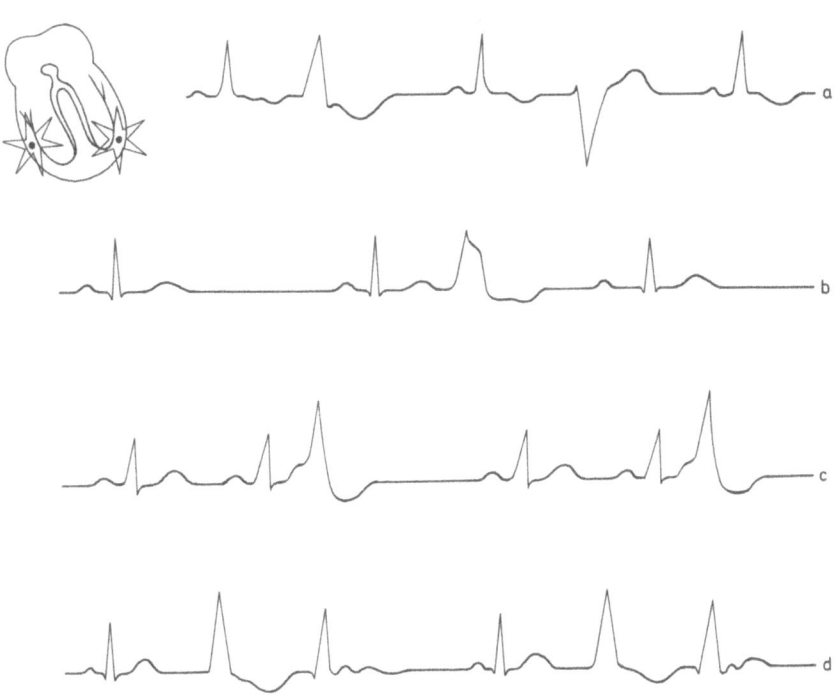

Fig. 87a–d. Ventricular extrasystoles. a) Right and left ventricular interpolated extrasystole. b) Interpolated extrasystole of right ventricular origin with PR prolongation before the ensuing normal beat (the conduction system is still depressed). c) Right ventricular extrasystole with compensatory pause (2:1 extrasystole, clinically: "trigeminy"). R on T phenomenon. d) Each normal beat is followed by two ventricular extrasystoles (clinically also manifest as "trigeminy")

Interpolated extrasystoles. They occur between two normal beats in such a manner that they do not disturb the slow basic rhythm and therefore appear without compensatory pause. The depolarization of the ensuing normal beat from the sinus node enters after the refractory phase of the extrasystole is over.

12.6.2 Escape Beats

In contrast to an extrasystole an escape beat appears belatedly in the cycle. Its interval from the previous normal beat is longer, if it is an extrasystole shorter, than the normal RR interval. Escape beats only occur in bradycardiac rhythms and they thus increase an otherwise hemodynamically unfavorable heart rate. — Passive heterotopy.

12.6.3 Escape Rhythms

The specific rhythms of secondary or tertiary impulse initiating centers (mentioned with the sinoatrial and atrioventricular types of block) can occur as *escape rhythms* (passive heterotopy) even without block, if the basic rhythm becomes too slow or ceases altogether.

Supraventricular escape rhythms usually originate in the bundle of His with a regular frequency of 40–60 per minute. Also, the QRS complexes are not altered because the ventricles are depolarized along the normal route. However, they may be slightly deformed by "aberrant conduction." These deformed but regular ventricular complexes are still recognizable as nodal rhythm in the presence of atrial fibrillation or flutter (Fig. 78, p. 107).

The *nodal rhythms* (His bundle rhythms) shown in Fig. 88 are diagnosed without difficulty if the negative P waves appearing before or after the ventricular complexes (due to retrograde stimulation of the atrium from the AV node) are clearly recognizable. But retrograde atrial stimulation does not necessarily occur (Fig. 88 a). If atrial and ventricular stimulation coincides, the negative P wave merges with the QRS complex (Fig. 88 c).

Ventricular escape rhythms have a rate of 20–40 per minute. The QRS and ST-T deflections are those of a bundle branch block — analogous to ventricular extrasystoles. In both cases the rule applies that right ventricular rhythms (and extrasystoles) look like left bundle branch block, left ventricular rhythms (and extrasystoles) like right bundle branch block. If an escape rhythm does not set in for several seconds this preautomatic pause results in Stokes-Adams attack.

Reentry mechanisms

Active heterotopic rhythms. In principle these are caused by focal stimuli or circuit stimulation (reentry mechanisms).

Disorders in the conduction system may lead to extrasystoles or ventricular tachycardia by a unidirectional block with reentry mechanism. It was shown experimentally that an injured branch may extinguish regular activation by a unidirectional block (branch B in Fig. 89), whereas slowed retrograde conduction is still feasible. If the muscle fiber M is reached via bundle A, retrograde conduction can take place via B. With adequate delay it reaches the bifurcation X when it is out of the refractory period and causes renewed depolarization of conduction and functional musculature (extrasystole). This can maintain the idioventricular tachycardia if "circus" stimulation continues.

Paroxysmal tachycardia is diagnosed when the sudden start can be ascertained in the history or by ECG. The attack may last from seconds or minutes to many days. Paroxysmal tachycardia

According to the origin of the impulse, supraventricular and ventricular tachycardia are distinguished and diagnosed chiefly by the shape of the ventricular complexes — in analogy to the extrasystoles.

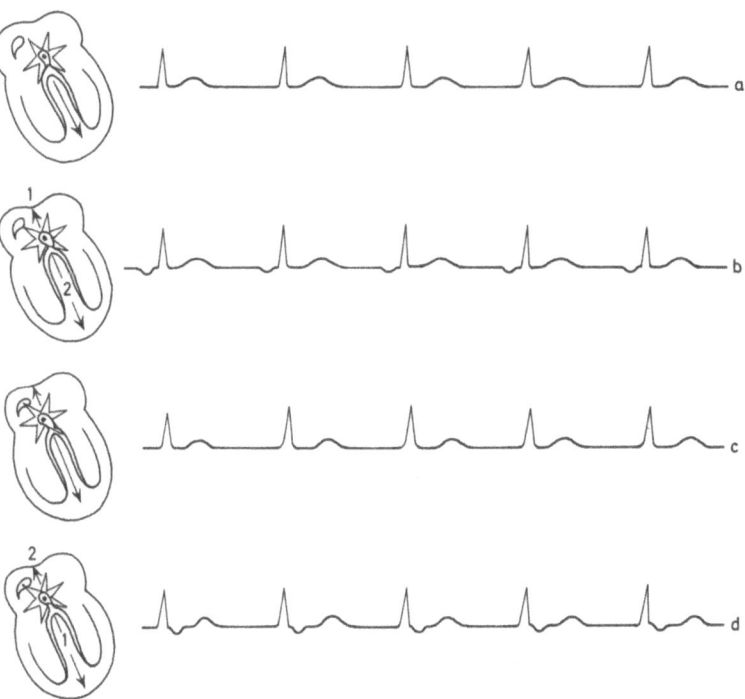

Fig. 88a–d. AV nodal rhythm. a) Without retrograde stimulation of atria. b) So-called upper nodal rhythm, where the atria (1) are activated retrogradely before the ventricles (2). c) So-called middle nodal rhythm, where atria and ventricles are activated simultaneously. d) So-called lower nodal rhythm, where the ventricles (1) are activated before the atria (2)

119

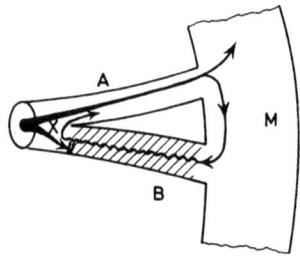

Fig. 89.   Diagram of re-entry mechanism.
Cause: circuit stimulation

Supraventricular tachycardias have a rate of between 120 and 250 per minute. A more exact localization of the ectopic focus in the atrium is feasible if formal differentiation of the P waves from the atrial waves of the normal rhythm can be made during an attack. In *paroxysmal sinus tachycardia*, the P waves are identical before and during the attack. In the more common *paroxysmal atrial tachycardia,* the ectopic focus arises in cranial segments of the atrium, the P waves are positive, but markedly deformed. In *paroxysmal nodal tachycardia* (focus in the bundle of His), negative P waves are seen — in analogy to the nodal rhythms — in leads II, III, aVF less than 0.12 s prior to or immediately after the ventricular complexes, or they are concealed in these. However, if the negative P wave appears more than 0.12 s ahead of the QRS complex, it is a *coronary sinus tachycardia.*

Clinically important is the recognition of *paroxysmal atrial tachycardia with AV block,* since it is mostly due to digitalis toxicity together with hypokalemia (Fig. 90). The atrial rate lies between 120 and 280 per minute, the AV block may be first-, second-, or third degree. In complete AV block there is usually a rapid AV nodal escape rhythm. Frequently, this type of atrial tachycardia does not start with paroxysms.

Not infrequently, paroxysmal tachycardia conceals paroxysmal atrial fibrillation or flutter.

The prognostically graver *paroxysmal ventricular tachycardia* occurs, in contradistinction to supraventricular tachycardia more often as an extrasystolic (Gallavardin) (Fig. 91) than as an essential (Bouveret-Hoffmann) type; that is, it starts and ends with increased ventricular extrasystoles that occur in bursts. The rate is 150–250 per minute. The beat sequence is usually not quite regular. The ventricular complexes are highly polymorphic at times (ventricular anarchy) and resemble bundle branch block in accordance with their ventricular origin. The side of the focus can be determined from their morphology analogous to the ventricular extrasystoles. Since retrograde conduction to the atria is almost always blocked, the undisturbed activity of the atria in sinus rhythm is recognized by interpersed P waves without relation to ventricular complexes. This observation permits reliable differentiation from supraventricular tachycardia with additional bundle branch block. Combined beats occur.

120

In the ECG differentiation of supraventricular tachycardia with a bundle branch block pattern of QRS complexes (ventricular aberration) from ventricular tachycardia, the following criteria have been offered in favor of a *supra*ventricular origin of the tachycardia:

Constant P-QRS relation

Right bundle branch block, type rsR′ in V1

Identical QRS complexes or identical initial vectors (0.04 s) as compared with the ECG at rest

Start of tachycardia with an extrasystolic P wave

This differentiation has the same therapeutic consequences as that of atrial fibrillation with aberrant spread of activation from interspersed extrasystoles. In the first case (aberrant spread of activation), additional digitalization is often indicated; in the second case (ventricular extrasystoles or tachycardia), it is life-threatening under certain conditions.

Frequently, transition from ventricular tachycardia to *ventricular flutter* is ill-defined. The ectopic rhythm develops an ever more rapid rate (200–300 per minute) and the tracing reveals uniform, large oscillations (hairpin curve), where main and terminal deflections can no longer be differentiated (Fig. 92).

In contrast, *ventricular fibrillation* display extremely rapid potential fluctuations of rate, shape, and amplitude, which no longer allow a hemodynamically effective cardiac contraction. The patient becomes unconscious; this is the tachysystolic or hyperdynamic type of the Stokes-Adams syndrome (Fig. 93).

12.6.4 Parasystoles (Para-arrhythmia)

The competition of two or several autonomous centers is known as *para-arrhythmia*. Whereas fixed coupling to the preceding normal excitation was mentioned with the extrasystoles (e.g., as bigeminy, a "twin pulse"), in para-arrhythmia, a second pacemaker located supraventricularly or ventricularly becomes active temporarily, independent of the sinus rhythm.

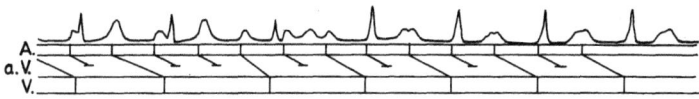

Fig. 90. Paroxysmal atrial tachycardia with AV block

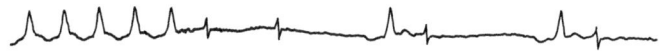

Fig. 91. Paroxysmal extrasystolic ventricular tachycardia

Ventricular flutter

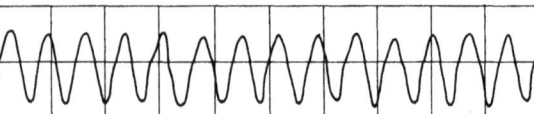

Fig. 92.   Ventricular flutter

Ventricular fibrillation

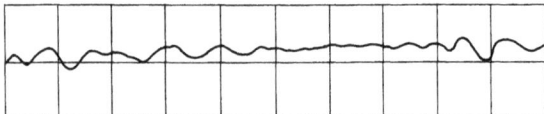

Fig. 93.   Ventricullar fibrillation

<table>
</table>

Simple AV dissociation

Simple AV dissociation (Fig. 94) arises if — without AV conduction disturbance — the specific rate of the sinus node declines transitorily below that of the AV node, e. g., as a sequel to sinus arrhythmia. A change follows between normally transmitted cardiac activation and a dissociation of atrial and ectopic ventricular function. The PR interval is not constant: apart from a normal PR interval, abnormal short intervals are found (apparent conduction only), or the P wave is superposed by the QRS complex or follows it.

Basically, this arrhythmia presents an intermittent AV nodal rhythm that occurs as a passive ectopic rhythm when the sinus rhythm attains a rate that is lower than the specific rate of the nodal rhythm.

Complete AV dissociation

A special type of AV dissociation is complete or *isorhythmic dissociation*, where atria and ventricles beat in dissociation for a prolonged period due to only little differences in sinus and AV rates. Sinus rhythm and specific nodal rhythm not rarely have a tendency to become adapted (synchronization). Ortho- or retrograde conduction could occur in this case but does not just because of the refractory phase.

Interference dissociation

In an AV dissociation with interference *(interference dissociation)* (Fig. 95) there is a twin automatism with an incomplete AV block which makes occasional orthograde, rarely retrograde, conduction possible. This type of para-arrhythmia is mostly observed when a secondary or tertiary autonomous center "fires" more rapidly than the sinus node, and the AV dissociation is interrupted occasionally or repeatedly by conduction: a sequence called interference. It is seen in digitalis toxicity. The essential sign in the differential diagnosis is demonstration of a protective block at the AV level, which constantly screens *one* of the two

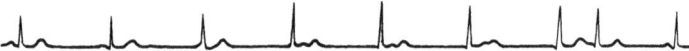

Fig. 94.   Simple AV dissociation

autonomous centers and here prevents extinction of activation due to the activity of the competing center.

Parasystole (Fig. 96) is a rare type of para-arrhythmia, in which two Parasystole different impulse-generating foci remain continuously active without cancelling each other out (both protectively blocked). On the one hand, the ventricles are controlled by the sinus rhythm or atrial fibrillation, but are also subject to a second slower parasystolic impulse center. This is protected by an entry block, develops a constant and indestructible idiorhythm; but it can act as pacemaker only — and becomes visible in the tracing — when its discharge occurs outside the refractory phase of the ventricles. Retrograde activation of the atria by the parasystolic center does not take place, so that the supraventricular center is protectively blocked in this way also. If the parasystoles are only irregularly interspersed in the tracing, they reveal a unifocal morphology which corresponds with their origin of excitation, but they always change intervals from the preceding conducting ventricular complexes (no fixed coupling!), as well as constant and divisible intervals.

In patients with a fixed-frequency pacemaker parasystoles are relatively frequent, if no complete AV block exists (any longer). Two types of excitation are in competition: one, arising from the sinus node (or atrial fibrillation) and one artificial, i. e., the one produced by the pacemaker electrode in a ventricle. Refractory conditions determine whether the natural or the artificial stimulus leads to spread of the activation.

12.7 Incidence of Different Types of Arrhythmia

According to an investigation by Katz (1963) on 6000 patients, the following types of arrhythmia were encountered: sinus arrhythmia (almost 100%), sinus tachycardia (3000), extrasystole (2000), atrial fibrillation (around 1500), sinus bradycardia (approx. 1000), AV block (about 800), rare disorders (about 500), atrial flutter (approximately 100).

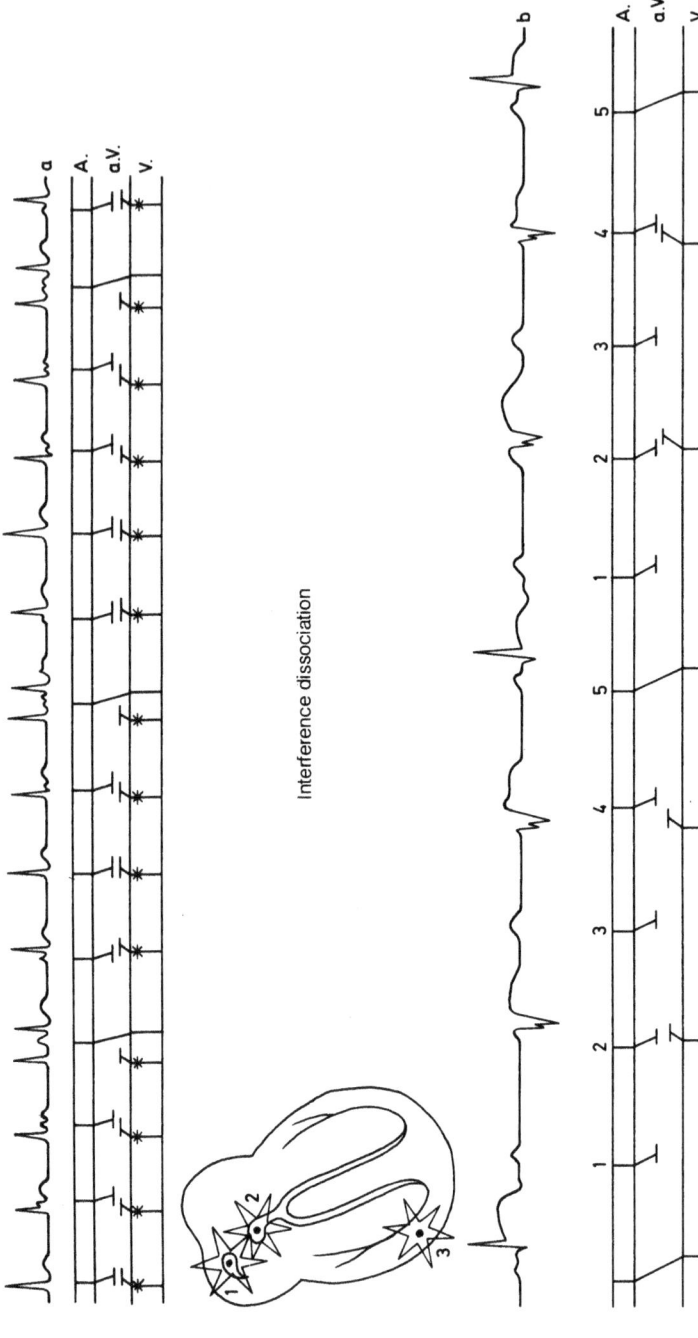

Interference dissociation

Fig. 95a and b. Interference dissociation. a) Apart from a sinus rhythm of the atria (1) there is a more rapid His bundle rhythm (2) of the ventricles, which leads to an AV dissociation. The QRS complexes 5, 10, 16 are of supraventricular origin (interference). The para-rhythm is thus temporarily disturbed (paracenter not protectively blocked). No retrograde conduction to atria (protective block). — Active heterotopy. b) Second-degree AV block, type 2 with 5:1 conduction. Ventricular escape rhythm from a right ventricular center (3), which leads to an AV dissociation. Each conduction (interference) disturbs the pararhythm temporarily. — Passive heterotopy

124

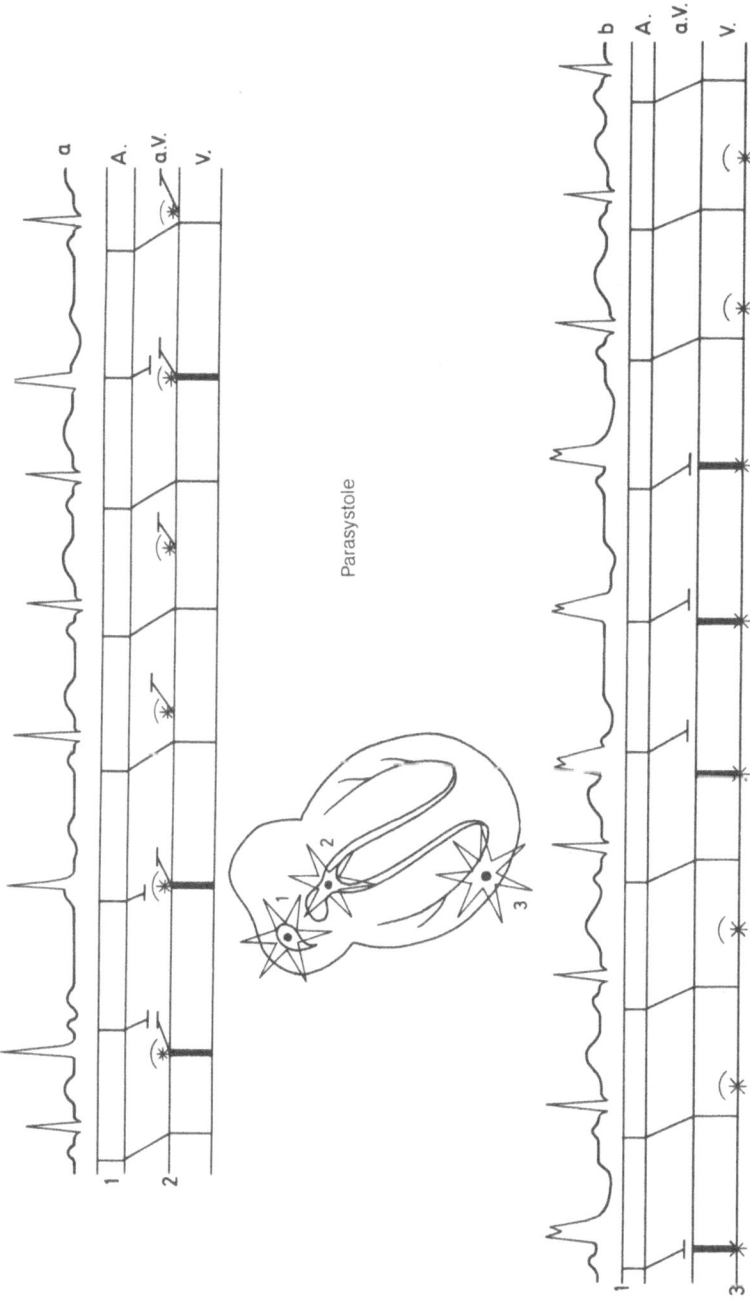

Parasystole

Fig. 96a and b. Parasystole. a) The parasystolic center is situated in the AV node (2). It produces an AV rhythm, which appears intermittently in the "false extrasystoles"; it remains silent only if its action falls in the refractory phase after previous normal ventricular stimulation. Its continuous and undisturbed (protectively blocked) activity can be demonstrated with dividers. No retrograde atrial activation (retrograde protective block at AV level). b) Parasystolic center (3) in ventricle

125

13. Pacemaker ECG

The impulse generator of an artificial pacemaker produces a spike-like deflection in the ECG with an impulse duration of 1.5–2 ms. If this impulse is ineffective, the spike is not followed by a ventricular complex. If the pacemaker impulse is effective, a typical spike is followed immediately by a deformed QRS complex which resembles a bundle branch block. According to the position of the stimulating electrode, the QRS complex resembles a left or a right bundle branch block. With most pacemakers in use today the stimulus is delivered by a transvenously introduced electrode in the right ventricle and thus causes QRS deformation of left bundle branch block type. This is similar to a ventricular automatism in which the stimulus originates in the right ventricle. If the active electrode has been fixed transthoracically to the left ventricle (as was the case in the early days of pacemaker therapy) by suturing the wires from a fixed-rate pacemaker to the epicardium of the left heart, then activation of the left ventricle is rapid and that of the right ventricle slowed. Therefore a right bundle branch block type QRS complex appears in the ECG after the pacemaker impulse spike, just as with ventricular automatism originating in the left ventricle.

Four kinds of pacemakers are available:

Fixed-rate pacemakers

Demand pacemakers

"R wave inhibited", (suppressed-demand, ventricular-inhibited)

"R wave triggered", (ventricular-triggered)

Atrial triggered pacemakers

Bifocal demand pacemakers

13.1 Fixed-Rate Pacemakers

With a fixed-rate pacemaker gradual recovery of sinus generation and AV stimulus conduction may lead to a parasystole, i. e., competition between the artificial and the physiologic pacemaker in the sinus node. This situation becomes highly dangerous if the pacemaker impulse falls into the vulnerable period of a spontaneous stimulation (cf. Fig. 87c, p. 117). Ventricular tachycardia and ventricular flutter may thus be provoked, though rarely. If the electric stimulation happens to fall in the period of physiologic AV conduction, a so-called combined systole (fusion beat) will result (Fig. 97).

13.2 Demand Pacemakers

Ventricle-regulated pacemakers give a stimulus only when the spontaneous heart rate declines below a pre-set rate (usually around 70).

13.2.1 R-Wave Inhibited

With an R-wave-blocked (inhibited) pacemaker the pacemaker impulses are suppressed by the "normal" QRS complexes, if their intrinsic rate is greater than that of the pacemaker. The demand pacemaker acts only if a sinus impulse does not arrive in the ventricle within the pre-set interval (Fig. 97).

13.2.2 R-Wave Triggered

With an R-wave-synchronized pacemaker an impulse is sent to the heart from a trigger unit with every R wave. If no QRS signal is received by the pacemaker, it stimulates at a fixed rate.

13.3 Atrial Triggered Pacemakers

An atrial-triggered pacemaker, which synchronizes atrial and ventricular action, would be particularly favorable hemodynamically, above all because it allows physiologic adaptation of the rate to physical effort. But it makes sense only in isolated AV conduction defects, i. e., not in the presence of co-existent abnormal sinoatrial activation or ectopic atrial activation, e. g., atrial fibrillation, which is not infrequently encountered in the elderly patient. (A disadvantage is its technical complexity and the need for thoracotomy to place the wires.)

13.4 Bifocal Demand Pacemakers

In bifocal demand pacemakers one stimulating electrode lies in the atrium and another in the ventricle. In sinus bradycardia, sinoatrial block, or sinus arrest with preserved AV conduction, only the atrium is stimulated (Fig. 97). If an AV block is present at the same time, the atrium, and after an appropriate AV interval also the ventricle, is stimulated. Spontaneous ventricular depolarization interrupts the fixed sequence of stimulation.

Examples of these types of pacemakers are given in Fig. 97 a–f.

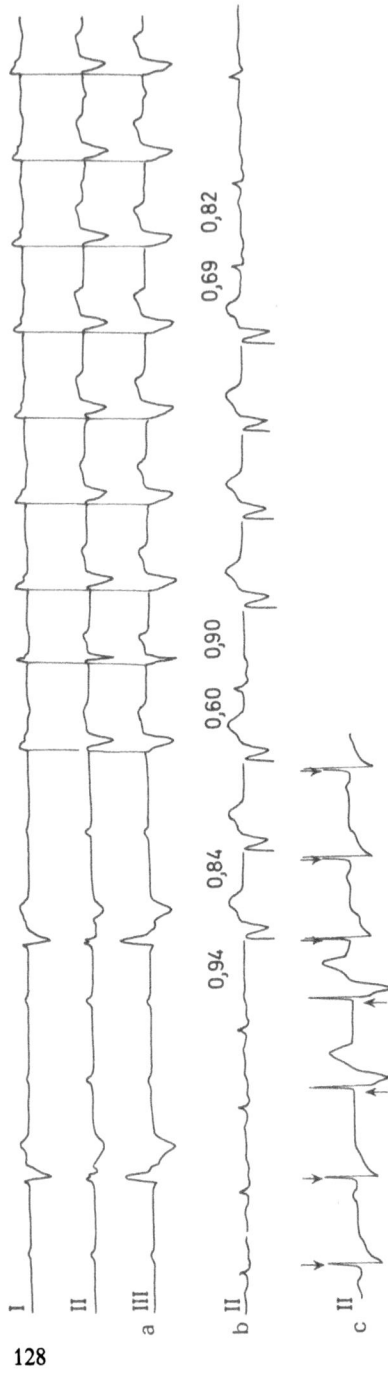

Fig. 97. a) Fixed-rate pacemaker. Implantation because of third-degree AV block with ventricular bradycardia. b) Demand pacemaker: no stimulation until absence of sinus activity for 0.94 s. Brief block of pacemaker impulses because of single spontaneous action, followed by renewed pacemaker discharge because of asystole. c) QRS synchronized demand program. Each R wave is followed by a pacemaker impulse which however, remains ineffective (↓). During a brief delay in sinus node discharge the pacemaker takes over (↑). d) Bifocal pacemaker stimulation. Atria and ventricles follow artificial stimulations in simulated natural sequence. e) Atrium-triggered ventricular stimulation. The natural atrial stimulation is followed after 0.14 s by the pacemaker impulse which activates the ventricle. f) Atrial stimulation. Atrial impulses are generated by an atrial electrode and transmitted to the ventricles

128

13.5 Complications After Pacemaker Implantation

13.5.1 Complete Failure of Pacemaker Impulses

In this case, there are no spikes in the ECG. The cause may be a broken electrode, for instance.

13.5.2 Normal Pacemaker Impulses Without Stimulus Response

The spikes are not followed by a QRS of bundle branch block pattern. This occurs when the contact of the pacemaker electrode with the endocardium is interrupted by dislocation of the electrode, or when the stimulus threshold is raised, as occurs occasionally after pacemaker implantation (exit block).

13.5.3 Racing Pacemaker

Incipient failure of an electrical pacemaker is recognized in the ECG by sudden, marked decrease or increase in the pacemaker rate. Since the frequent pacemaker impulses may be transmitted to the ventricles and cause a response, the ECG reveals a high ventricular rate, e. g., 150 per minute. This can have serious hemodynamic consequences. An approximate guide is an increase or decrease in pacemaker rate of 5% of the initially set value. These changes in rate are indicators of exhaustion of the energy supply of the pacemaker which requires exchange.

14. ECG in Children*

Many factors that have to be considered in ECG diagnosis of adults (e. g., degenerative diseases of the heart, toxic effects of drugs, nicotine, etc.) play practically no part in childhood, and hence conditions appear less complicated. But correct evaluation of tracings of children can prove difficult even to the experienced. The reasons may be summarized in the following points:

Why is evaluation of the childhood ECG difficult?

The brief physiologic *devolution of the ECG* requires knowledge of the normal values for each age group. However, the normal range varies greatly.

The *configuration* of ECG tracings *peculiar* to children may be unfamiliar to a doctor predominantly working in adult cardiology.

Extracardiac factors play a much greater part in children than in adults; they vary from age group to age group and, are often difficult to differentiate.

Recording of faultless tracings meets with purely *technical difficulties,* especially in young children: artifacts due to restlessness, crying, slipping of electrodes, etc., must be taken account of in interpretation.

14.1 Normal Development of ECG as a Whole

14.1.1 Newborns

The fetal heart resembles a "double pump" interpolated into the systemic circulation. The aorta is supplied with blood from the left – via the physiologic shunts through the foramen ovale and ductus arteriosus – and from the right heart in approximately equal proportions. This "dynamic equilibrium" results anatomically in the characteristic *balance of mass* of the two halves of the heart of a newborn. The muscle mass ratio right to left is approximately 1 : 1 in the newborn, in the adult 1 : 2.6. In the newborn, the right ventricle is thus more than twice as heavy as the left when compared with the left ventricle of the adult.

"Physiologic right hypertrophy" of the newborn

Hence, it is justifiable to speak of a *"physiologic right hypertrophy"* of neonates.

Thus, the ECG of the newborn reveals right axis deviation (up to +180°), deep S in leads I and aVL, tall R in leads III, aVF, and usually also in aVR. In the chest leads there are tall positive deflections over the right (R in V3r, V1, V2), deep negative waves over the left precordium (S in V5, V6).

---

* By P. Schumacher

The preponderance of the right ventricle is especially impressive in the vectorcardiogram (Fig. 98). The vector loop of the newborn lies almost completely to the right of the vector origin, both in the frontal and horizontal projections, and thus represents almost the mirror image of that commonly seen in adults. The vector loop reveals at first glance that most vectors run toward the right leads (V1, V2, III, aVR). This explains the tall R waves in these leads as well as the deep S waves in all leads over the left of the heart (V5, V6, I, aVL).

During the first weeks of life the vector loop in the horizontal projection is inscribed in a direction (clockwise) opposite to that of the later normal one (anticlockwise) (see *arrow* in Fig. 98). As a result of this different vector rotation there is normally in the newborn a relative prolongation of the QR interval over the right chest with simultaneous shortening over the left. The positive difference QR in V6–QR in V1 of the older child is thus negative in the majoritiy of neonates.

14.1.2 Infants

A transition from a few hours to days is required for the fetal circulation to adapt to postfetal conditions. This process varies considerably in time but is basically quite regular on ECG and continues into adulthood. Due to altered hemodynamic conditions in the first few months of life the structure of the heart is transformed. The left ventricle increasingly dominates in supplying the systemic circulation, whereas the right ventricle undergoes a kind of "physiologic atrophy."

Regression of right preponderance

The strengthening of the left ventricle is reflected mainly in the left chest leads. The small neonatal R in V5. V6 rapidly becomes larger, the S wave correspondingly smaller. After a few months the QRS complexes in the left chest leads hardly differ from those seen at a later age. In the right chest leads (V1, V2), the signs of right preponderance also regress distinctly (R becomes smaller, S deeper), but not as fast as in the left leads. An R in V1 and V2, relatively tall as compared with the adult norm, persists throughout childhood (Fig. 98).

14.1.3 Young Children

At the end of the first year of life the structural change in the heart is usually completed, and the normal mass relation of the ventricles has been almost attained. Growth-induced change in the position of the heart within the thorax now occurs and is affected by different factors in the different age groups.

The *anatomic transverse position* of the heart in the first few years is due to the relatively large transverse and small vertical diameter of the thorax together with the physiologically raised diaphragm. Contrary to adult conditions, the right ventricle occupies a far greater proportion of the anterior surface of the heart, which appears to be rotated clockwise on its longitudinal axis. Wheras the horizontal position of the infant heart is electrically fully compensated by the vector projection resulting from muscle-mass relationships and cannot be seen in the ECG, rotation on the longitudinal axis is manifest by an extremely deep *Q wave in lead III* which is typical of early childhood. A depth of Q in excess of the accepted adult threshold of 25% of the height of the R wave is almost the

Deep Q3

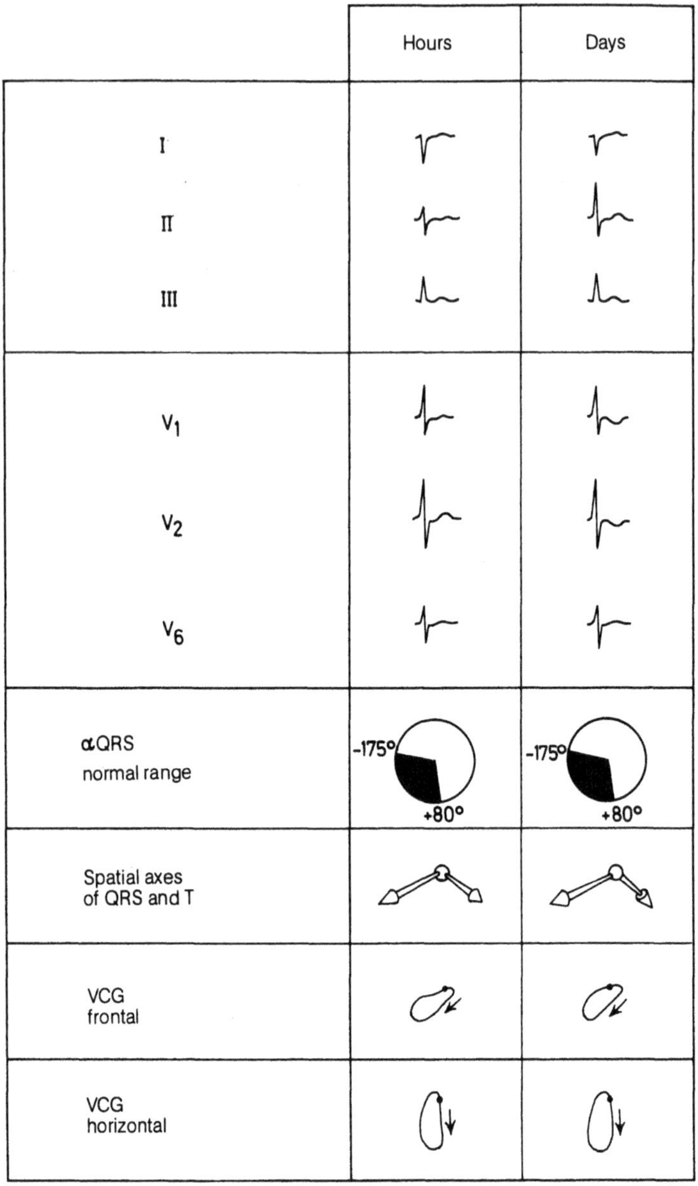
Hours
Days
I
II
III
V1
V2
V6
αQRS
normal range
-175°
+80°
-175°
+80°
Spatial axes
of QRS and T
VCG
frontal
VCG
horizontal

a

Fig. 98a and b. Development of the ECG in children

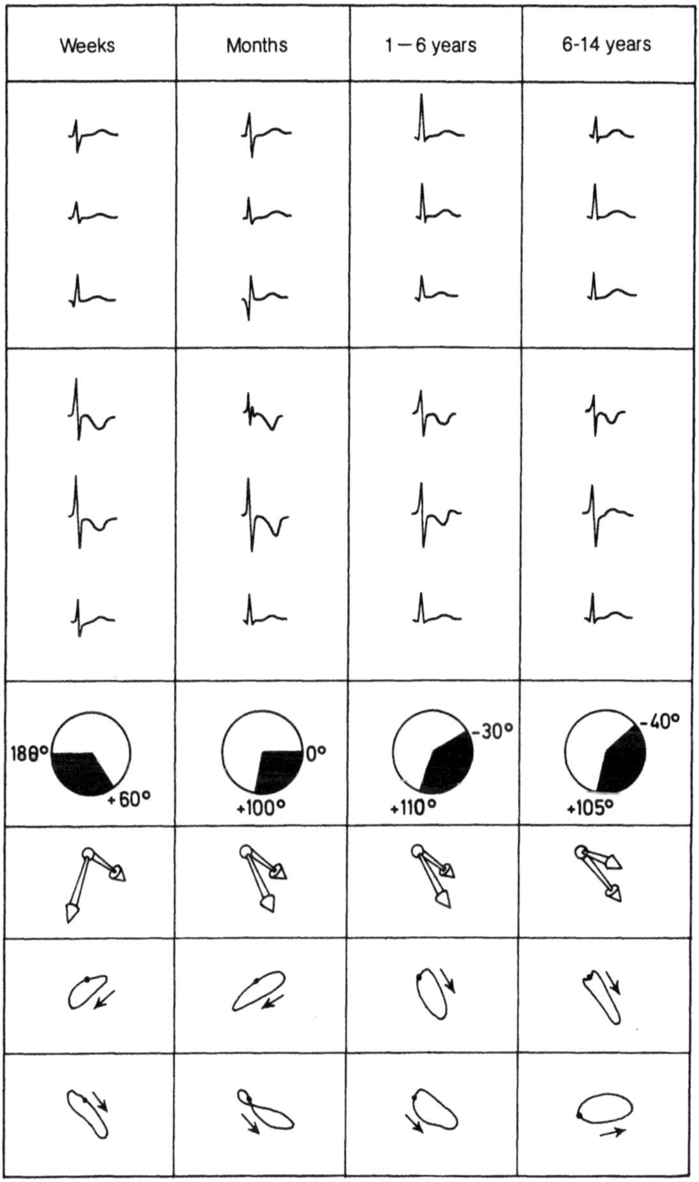

Weeks	Months	1 — 6 years	6-14 years

b

Fig. 98. (continued)

133

rule in Q 3 of the young infant; it may even become the largest deflection of the QRS complex without being pathologic.

Along with the gradual regression of the physiologic right ventricular hypertrophy, the anatomic transverse position of the heart may be reflected in the ECG and cause occasional diagnostic difficulties. Whereas marked left axis deviation in the infant ECG has to be regarded as pathologic or at least as an important indicator to an abnormal process in the heart (e. g., congenital tricuspid stenosis), axis positions below 30° are not infrequent in children with normal hearts in the second and third years. This ranges from a marked R1 S3 type indicating transverse position to an S1 Q3 type following rotation round the longitudinal axis in young children.

R is already dominant in the left precordial leads (V5, V6), but the predominant S of adults over the right precordium is not so distinct as yet.

Left axis deviation of small children

14.1.4 School-Aged Children

Increased longitudinal growth beginning with the fourth to sixth year, concomitant with an increase in the vertical thoracic diameter, stretches the mediastinum, so to speak, at school age. The heart rotates around the sagittal axis to the right, with gradual compensation of rotation on the longitudinal axis. The resulting anatomic and electric vertical position of the heart produces the characteristic ECG of the older child and adolescent: the r1R3 to S1R3 type. The electric position is vertical (rS in aVL, qR in aVF) to semivertical. In the chest leads, S is already preponderant over the right precordium, but the R wave is frequently still higher than the adult norm.

Apart from the typical features of childhood tracings, the ECG time limits are also characteristic. Table 6 lists in a simplified manner the most important upper limits at different ages. For special cases the normal values applicable to each age should be obtained from one of the many statistical tables available. For daily practice the memorizing of a few simplified maximal values is adequate.

Table 6. Simplified upper-limit values of the infant ECG at different ages.

	Infant	Small child	School child
P duration:	0.07 s	0.08 s	0.09 s
P height:	2.5 mm	3 mm	3 mm
AV interval:	0.15 s	0.17 s	0.19 s
QRS duration:	0.07 s	0.08 s	0.09 s

14.2 Morphologic Characteristic Patterns of Childhood Tracings

P wave: Apart from a considerable variety of shapes — mainly due to extracardiac factors which will be discussed later — the P wave of the child differs only slightly from that of the adult. Typical of the *newborn* ECG is a tall and peaked P, especially in leads II and III (P pulmonale) in a high percentage of cases. It is probably based on adaptation processes to postfetal conditions in the course of temporary overloading of the right heart; it regresses within a few days.

A negative P wave in lead III, not uncommon in children of school age, may be misinterpreted. This finding is remarkable, since — with the vertical axis of the older child — the corresponding QRS group is predominantly directed upward, i. e., discordant to the P wave. The cause of the divergence of the P vector from the QRS axis, hardly observed in healthy adults, is probably a lower-lying impulse origin at the tail end of the sinus node. Thus, spread of the stimulation in the atria will adopt a more horizontal course even from below upward. This finding must not be thought of as pathologic. If it were an AV rhythm significant shortening of the AV interval would have to be present as well. `Negative P3`

The *AV interval* (PR interval) in children is naturally shorter than in adults and rises more or less continuously from birth to puberty (for upper limits, see Table 6). It is important to know that values below 0.1 s in infants and young children are quite normal and do not indicate an ectopic origin or pathologically shortened conduction, as they would in adults. `PR interval less than 0.1 s`

QRS complex: Apart from the specific relationships of the different waves, some further peculiarities of the QRS group in childhood should be metioned: the *amplitudes* of the individual deflections of the limb leads are frequently smaller in infants than at a later age, but already reach almost normal adult values in small children. Conditions differ for chest leads, where much higher deflections are written, because of the thin chest wall and the close approximation of the heart to it, than in adults. Amplitudes of several mV are found, especially left parasternally, a fact that ought not to mislead to a rash diagnosis of ventricular hypertrophy. `High QRS amplitudes in chest leads`

(The difficult ECG diagnosis of hypertrophy in childhood cannot be discussed in detail in a short introduction. However, it may be mentioned that various indices calculated from wave amplitudes can be applied to children only if much modified.)

The shape of the QRS complex in children is as a rule slim, but slurring and notching is common and of the same significance as in adults. Special differential diagnostic difficulties are caused by the M shape of the QRS complex in the right chest leads (V3r, V1, V2), a finding still generally called *"incomplete right bundle branch block"*, `RR' configuration over the right chest wall` although conduction delay in the right ventricular branch is only one of many possibilities. In the child, an RR' complex over the right chest wall may indeed indicate right ventricular hypertrophy or overloading; or it may occur in the course of a myocarditis and be the sole ECG sign of disease. In funnel chest it can indicate extreme rightward rotation of the heart, but in the majority of cases it is a diagnostically and prognostically harmless variant of the vector projection which is typical in children. Practically all criteria for its differential diagnosis in adults, also called "physiologic right bundle branch block", from its pathologic forms are of no help in children. An approximate distinction can be made only by careful consideration of the whole ECG and clinical picture (e. g., other signs of hypertrophy, lengthened PR indicating simultaneous myocarditis, etc.).

In general it can be said that discovery of a pathologic cause in childhood is the exception rather than the rule. There should be no hesitation when assessing an ECG. It would be quite wrong to mention ECG changes, to the patient or his parents in the absence of abnormal clinical findings. Parental apprehension will be of no benefit to the child.

Also, in a written report, the term "incomplete right bundle branch block" should be reserved for definitely abnormal forms. It is preferable to speak noncommittally of an RR' configuration or an M shape of the QRS complex over the right precordium.

ST displacement *ST-T segment:* Apart from a nonpathologic elevation above the zero line, seen in the first 3–4 weeks of life, the ST-T segments do not show any typical changes in childhood. As will be explained below, deviation of more than 0.1 mV from the isoelectric line is no longer normal in children either, although the percentage distribution of the many causes differs from that of adults.

Negative T over the right chest *T wave:* It is the T waves which display the greatest differences from those in adults. As a rule, their typical pattern in the chest leads permits recognition at first glance that a child's tracing is being looked at. Ignorance of these characteristics leads to grave errors.

For reasons as yet unknown, the spatial T vector in children points posteriorly to the left and only gradually rotates to its later normal anterior left position. (Fig. 98).

Therefore, in contrast to adults, the T wave of children is *negative* over a large part of the chest wall. During further development the negativity gradually moves to the right and may persist over the right chest wall (V3r, V1) into adolescence. Nevertheless, the T waves of the newborn occupy a special position which (presumably due to a temporary increase in pressure in the right heart) can be positive over the right and isolectric to negative over the left chest wall. This behavior, also called "physiologic myocardial injury of the newborn" is observed in the limb leads by a general flattening up to inversion of the T waves. It is taken as a sign of adaptation to the completely changed hemodynamic situation from that of the fetus. At the latest this adaptive phase has been overcome at the end of the first week of life, so that positive T waves over the right precordium have to be regarded as repolarization defects throughout childhood up to the tenth or twelfth year.

Table 7 lists the progressive rightward shift of a negative T with increasing age by indicating the age limits at which a negative or diphasic T wave can still be considered normal.

In addition to its direction, the shape of the ST-T segment over the right precordium frequently diverges considerably in children from the usual pattern in adults. A preterminally negative T wave, arising from a depressed, upward convex ST-T segment is very common and it often ends only in a very slight terminal positive phase. This typical childhood pattern, also called "childhood T", is quite normal. It must not be "Child-interpreted as a sign of hypertrophy or abnormal right ventricular hood T" repolarization , despite its overt resemblance to the described "hypertrophic form" or the "roller coaster" curve.

Frequently, distinctly diphasic T waves are found, predominantly in the transition zone, of quite bizarre shapes. Double peaks are also quite normal.

Table 7. Patterns of T waves in chest leads of children.
The figures refer to the age up to which negative or diphasic T waves in the different leads can still be regarded as normal (modified after Ziegler)

	T negative	T diphasic
V1	Normal to adolescence	
V2	Up to 12 years	Up to 16 years
V3	Up to 10 years	Up to 15 years
V4	Up to 5 years	Up to 11 years
V5	Up to 15 h	Up to 14 h
V6	Up to 8 h	Up to 24 h

Apart from T changes in chest leads, T waves are often misinterpreted in lead III. Whereas in the adult a negative T3 is usually seen only in left axis deviation with a concordant negative main QRS deflection in lead Negative T3 III, a negative T3 is not uncommon in vertical or right axis deviation of children. At first glance this looks like a pathologic ST-T discordant to the QRS complex, but is diagnostically unimportant, unless a repolarization disorder is manifest in the remaining leads. Physiology and pathology factors in childhood must also be borne in mind when assessing the rather frequent "nonspecific" repolarization disorders (e. g., general flattening of T, ST depression, etc.). Whereas chronic degenerative processes and circulatory disorders prevail with increasing age, in childhood these are — apart from extracardiac effects — mainly acute, rapidly reversible changes in the myocardium, morbid-anatomically barely demonstrable — or of its electric response. It would be wrong to "condemn" a child to having myocardial damage on the basis of a single, apparently pathologic, finding: this would induce in the child a vicious circle of physical protection, awareness of being ill, etc.

14.3 Effects of Extracardiac Factors

Effects on tracings due to extracardiac mechanisms play a greater part throughout life than is generally supposed. (See chapter 10, Changes in ST-T segment). This applies to children, in the first instance. The dynamics of development associated with its many, not always harmonic growth processes and maturation of organ functions constantly provide fresh upsets of the overall metabolism. These affect the ECG also and in many cases are not easy to explain. Their influence in childhood and possible misinterpretation of juvenile tracings will be indicated here.

Labile metabolism of infants
Labile metabolism and ionic balance often affect the ECG of infants. Relatively minor nutritional disturbance, diarrhea, vomiting, etc., cause a rapid shift in pH and electrolytes. Flattening of T waves, displacement of ST-T segment, distinct U waves (hypokalemia), QT prolongation (hypocalcemia) may ensue.

"Anxiety ECG" of young children
In young children the above-mentioned *changes in position of the thoracic organs* due to growth predominate. But even then, mental factors supervene whose significance is easily underestimated. The understandable *anxiety* of a child faced with examination, apparatus and uncommon surroundings may simulate a pathologic ECG with ST depression and T flattening. Only a repeat ECG when the child is in a calm frame of mind or asleep evinces the true situation.

Two important lessons derive from this fact for ECG in children:
1: To obtain a useful ECG of a child requires time and patience. The child must have the opportunity to get accustomed to the doctor's room or ECG laboratory. Registering the strip ought to be a game rather than a procedure.

2. The doctor himself should be present during the recording, since he will thus be able to assess the psychologic reaction of the child, and errors may be prevented.

School age — particularly prepuberty and puberty — is characterized by a momentous *change in endocrine and autonomous nervous systems,* apart from purely physical growth. This period is rarely smooth and many inadequate reactions may be reflected in the ECG. Here also repolarization disturbances are typical but nonspecific. Almost every

Orthostatic syndrome
child reveals a more or less marked *orthostatic circulatory dysfunction.* This can still be observed, immediately after the child has lain down, by

ST depression, T flattening, even T inversion, and simulates a primary cardiac condition. In this case, full testing of cardiovascular functions should be added with an ECG recorded at rest, on standing, and on exercise. The lability of this age group is also manifest by clear *diurnal fluctuations*. It is not uncommon to obtain different tracings on different days or at different times of day. Diurnal fluctuations

Atrial depolarization appears to be especially dependent on autonomic nervous system effects. It is not surprising therefore, that the lability of the autonomic nervous system is evidenced by a *variable shape of the P wave* during prepuberty and puberty. Increase or decrease in amplitude, double peaks, or a lengthened P wave in one or several leads may alternate rapidly, and should not be labeled as pathologic in the absence of signs of disease. Labile P wave

The frequently negative P wave in lead III of children has been mentioned. In addition, mostly in prepuberty and puberty, a gradual or erratic change of direction of the P wave in lead III (less marked in lead II) is not uncommonly observed, the AV interval remaining constant or only minimally altered. This is a *wandering pacemaker* within the anatomically usually elongated sinus node which extends far distally. This change is also harmless and just reflects a labile autonomic nervous system.

The list of functional ECG changes found in prepuberty and puberty could be continued as desired. Atrial extrasystoles, partial AV block, AV rhythm, AV dissociation, etc., can occur and render diagnosis difficult. In principle, the clinical picture is decisive, and a diagnosis referring to the heart must never be made from the ECG alone. Indeed, the physiologic labile autonomic nervous system of the older child points to the responsibility carried by the physician: myocarditis, which can produce identical ECG changes, would demand physical rest and prohibition of gymnastics, athletics, sports, etc., as would a toxic-infectious disorder of the heart muscle. On the contrary, a child revealing autonomic nervous system imbalance and peripheral dysfunction should be encouraged to take physical exercise, as pampering would lead to deterioration. The common practice of being pessimistic with uncertain ECG findings and to advise physical caution "for safety" may be justified in adults; but abandoning gymnastics, sports, and games means restricting physical and mental development for the child. Incidence of autonomic ECG changes in prepuberty and puberty

14.4 Technical Difficulties

In addition to the functional effects on the ECG, external conditions can produce changes in the tracings of infants and young children that cause errors. Vibrations and fluctuations of the isoelectric line due to *physical restlessness* of the patient are generally known. Patience and friendly persuasion are supported by the milk bottle, a dummy, darkened room, or allowing the mother to hold the child. Occasionally, administration of a sedative (e. g., chloral hydrate per rectum, sodium pentobarbital suppositories, etc.) will be necessary. *Forced crying* causes (apart from muscle tremors) axis deviation of the heart in the thorax, and not rarely an RR' complex over the right precordium. Also, eructation, swallowing and particularly in infants, singultus, produce ECG distortion and waves that may be mistaken for extrasystoles.

Specially important for ECG during the entire childhood are the chest leads, which actually reflect cardiac electric processes much better than the limb leads, which are more affected by extracardiac factors. However, an exact technique adapted to the anatomic conditions of children is required.

The electrodes commonly used for adults may be employed during school age, but they would take up too large areas of the heart and produce unclear summation patterns in smaller children.

A suction electrode with a head of approximately 1 cm in diameter and a plug connection not directly at the electrode — in order to prevent it from tilting — but at the end of a 15 cm long intermediate cable, has been specially designed for infants and small children. Ordinary ECG electrodes can also be used, but must be fixed with adhesive plaster. A plain exploring electrode with a comparatively small head may suffice for single-channel recorders.

The points of placement of the various electrodes are the same for the older child as for the adult. In the infant, with its raised diaphragm and small vertical thoracic diameter, the heart lies somewhat higher. Hence, leads V4 to V6 should be placed in the 4th instead of in the 5th intercostal space.

The small size of the child's heart makes it obvious that already minor changes in electrode position result in considerable changes of ECG patterns. Serial tests entailing many checks are particularly important in childhood. Therefore, caution is indicated when changes occur during observation (e. g., in QRS amplitude) which can be due to negligible misplacement of an electrode.

Special care should be given to the sparse use of electrode paste, which must be applied only to the site of placement. The small distances between lead points favor short circuiting which would yield a completely distorted chest ECG.

15. Technique of ECG Recording*

The following brief guide to interference-free recording of ECGs requires equipment in good working order and screened cables for connecting the patient to the apparatus. Only those interferences will be discussed that arise from incompetent operation.

Difficulties during recording can be due to:

Interference from the alternating current

A wandering base line

Vibrating curve

Interference due to alternating current (AC) does not occur with battery equipment. Neither earthing wire nor charger must be connected with the ECG apparatus. Switching on of the charger is not enough — remove plug!

The causes of AC interference are voltage drops that build up on the skin of the patient during the flow of capacitively scattered current voltages from the electrodes in their course to the ground. They are inhibited by interruption of the earthing connection. It is true that the electrodes are exposed to capacitance interference also with battery-run ECG sets, but are compensated, since the apparatus receives the same alternating current impulses.

A lighting circuit with an AC of 220 V tension is common. But the action potentials of the heart muscle are maximally around values of 2 mV (millivolt). This 100,000-fold predominance must be guarded against. To make it still simpler for the "technical layman": it is the same as if a candlelight was to be seen near a sun lamp. In this case, the candlelight has to be screened from the glare of the sun lamp in order to be seen. Similarly, protection from the capacitance transmission of the 220,000 mV of the mains is achieved by registering an ECG in a screened chamber, the so-called Faraday cage. A Faraday cage consists of close-meshed metal net surrounding the whole room including windows and doors. It is connected with the earth potential (the waterpipes). Earth is always at zero potential, hence no interference can arise from it. But a Faraday cage can only be installed in scientific laboratories as it is very costly. In practice, other modes of suppression have to be employed. The zero potential of the earth (underground water) absolutely excludes any interference. But this underground water is reached only via the waterpipe as a ground connection, while central heating pipes often only

Alternating current interference

---

* By Wolfgang Newesely, Engineer

141

go as far as the boiler in the basement. As this may be filled using a hose now and then, it is not necessarily connected to the underground water.

The patient cable has five strands. One of them, attached to the right foot, connects the zero earth potential directly to the body of the patient via the ECG apparatus. The patient is thus grounded. He is at zero potential and cannot himself cause any capacitance AC interference. Despite the connection of the patient to the zero potential of the earth via the ground wire on the right leg, AC interference could still however be registered, if bringing all electrodes electrically close to the underground water zero potential were also unsuccessful. Only once the electrodes are at zero potential, no AC interference will take place. An important factor to be observed is that the skin, which has different insulating values, lies between the electrode and the interior of the body.

Skin resistance For instance, people working in the open and being suntanned have a much higher skin resistance than others. The skin resistance ranges between 5000 ohm and 200,000 ohm. The alternating current that has been received by capacitance from the electrodes has to overcome this skin resistance on its way to the zero potential via the body of the patient. According to Ohm's law, when an electric current flows through a resistor, a voltage drop develops which increases with the magnitude of the resistance to be overcome. This voltage drop of the interference is taken up by the electrodes and transmitted to the ECG apparatus. Thus it would be registered simultaneously with the myocardial action potential if all ECG sets were not constructed in such a manner that they eliminate disturbing voltages appearing at the electrodes in equal magnitude, equal phase, and at the same time. This elimination is possible only if the interfering voltages do not exceed many times over the values of the effective voltage derived from the patient.

It has just been stated that the apparatus can eliminate interferences only when it occurs at the electrodes in equal magnitude, equal phase, and synchronously. But the electrodes have different distances from interfering power circuits in the room. The electrode closest to the mains installation also receives a greater interfering voltage drop. As a result, different degrees of interfering potentials develop across the skin resistances. If the difference is only 0.001 V, an AC tracing of 1 mV is written. This corresponds to a curve width with the amplitude of the calibration mark. This obviously renders the tracing useless. The best protection from this type of interference is to reduce the skin resistance.

Reduction of skin resistance To begin with, the electrode jelly is rubbed into the skin with finger pressure. If this is unsuccessful, the skin is rubbed with moderately coarse glass paper. The insulating epidermis is thus removed and dermal circulation stimulated, which also diminishes resistance. Values of 200,000 ohm can be reduced by this harmless procedure to 5000–8000 ohm. These are relatively small amounts, the resulting decrease of interfering voltage drop is insignificant and the tracings are not affected. It must also be borne in mind that skin resistance depends on the size of

142

the electrode. The larger the electrode, the more is skin resistance reduced. However, the chest electrode is small in comparison to the limb electrode. Hence, interference is more frequent when recording chest leads than standard leads. If AC interference occurs only in chest leads and glass paper rubbing is not practicable, at least the electrode jelly must be rubbed in thoroughly. In very hairy patients lathering of the chest may help. The hairs are softened and the electrode is more easily attached. Finally, a remedy for AC interference may be mentioned: removal of the patient's bed from the wall and placing floor lamps, radios, bell wiring and mains cables to the ECG set far away from the patient. Reversing polarity of the power plug in the socket helps occasionally.

For orientation which limb electrode does not "fit electrically", the Goldberger leads should be switched on in series. If the tracing shows interference at aVR, the cause of the interference must be sought in the right arm. In aVL interference, the cause lies in the left arm. In case of aVF interference the left leg must be checked.

To ascertain whether mains voltage fluctuations exist which are not adequately equalized by the compensating circuit of the equipment, the following procedure should be adopted: Mains voltage fluctuation

Obtain three crocodile clips from a radio dealer and connect the plugs for right and left arms, and left foot (without patient!) by means of these clips. The written tracing ought to be a straight line under normal conditions (compensating circuit working properly) (switch position on lead I).

If two foils of different metal are dipped into a conducting fluid, a galvanic element is produced. According to the nature of the metal and dependent on the composition of the fluid (the electrolyte), this element produces a certain tension through polarization. The electrodes which have been applied to the patient by using a fluid (electrode jelly, soap or water) behave similarly. If the electrodes were to consist of the same material, no polarizing tension would result. Unfortunately this is impractical, and even minute impurities suffice to provoke polarization processes between the electrode plates. Basic fluids (soap, electrode jelly) cause fewer potentials than acid media. Hence, normal saline must never be used. If these electric potentials were to remain equal, they would not affect the tracing, since the wiring scheme in the apparatus is so arranged that direct current is not recorded as long as its magnitude does not change. But polarization processes need some time to become stabilized. A short period thus has to lapse after applying the electrodes before the tracing has become stable.

Despite these "small elements" that arise between apparatus and patient, faultless curves can still be written if there is no mechanical movement. If electrodes are not applied carefully or a pull is exerted on them by the patient cable, gross deviations of the baseline occur up and down even with respiration. These faults are particularly marked on Wandering of the baseline

143

chest leads. Hence the patient cable should not be allowed to hang down between equipment and electrodes. It is preferable to place the center of the cable (from where the five strands branch) on the patient's abdomen. At times it is necessary to ask the patient to stop breathing when recording the chest leads. In perspiring patients the sweat must be carefully neutralized to avoid electrolyte interference (washing with soap!). Some fabric should be placed as electrolyte carrier between the patient's skin and the electrode surface. It is helpful to have linen covers for the electrodes but they must be kept meticulously clean of course. Both linen and felt covers of the disk electrodes should be boiled in soda solution from time to time.

Vibration Vibrations can occur in the tracing (muscle tremors) if the patient does not relax completely. Apart from an agreeable room temperature, a wide comfortable couch is required for ECG. The patient's joints should be in an intermediate position (arms slightly flexed, a rolled blanket under the knees). This is especially important in the elderly. Some patients are alarmed before their first ECG when faced with the complicated electric equipment and need to be reassured by explaining to them that no electric current will affect them, but that only the current arising from their heart's activity is measured. Large rooms ought to be fitted with an infrared heater above the ECG couch. In general comfort is the keyword for successful ECG. Hence, it is also important that the temperature of the water with which the electrode covers are moistened is neither too high nor too low.

Finally, two methods will be mentioned by which proper functioning of the ECG equipment can be tested.

Equipment testing All sets having recording levers need to bridge frictional resistance between lever and paper. This renders writing of a double-peaked P or a small Q difficult. Slurring of R may also be lost.

In order to make sure that this important frictional resistance is not too great, a calibration mark of only 1 mm is recorded by turning down the sensitivity switch. In only very few cases will this "mini calibration trace" show the desired vertical rise from the baseline. Nevertheless, the registered pattern should still be a distinct trapezoid. A recorder that "forces itself" from the isoelectric position with a 1 mm/1 mV calibration trace will not make small potential differences visible.

Jet writers do not display this fault, since the ink jet has no friction.

The above check is also advisable for multiple recorders. Another important function test is to check uniformity of the calibration mark in all channels. Absolutely equal calibration signals of 1 cm must be written in all channels. In the Wilson leads one uses the one with the clearest deflection.

All chest plugs are now connected, directly or by means of alligator clips, to one chest electrode. Turning the switch from one lead to the other, identical curves must result. If one of them is too small, the calibration which normally should be 1 cm, is too large.

144

Tilting of the chest electrodes (by the apex beat) may cause distortion of the curve. To avoid this, suction electrodes are now available with plug and socket attached directly at the suction cup.

16. Concluding Cautionary Remarks on ECG Interpretation

Much uneasiness and disappointment of some doctors — amateurs in ECG — originates from their wrong approach to the possibilities and limitations of this diagnostic aid.

What is achieved by an ECG? The ECG is valuable in the diagnosis of the following cardiac conditions:

The arrhythmias

Infarction

Suspected hypertrophy of individual parts of the heart

16.1 Cardiac Arrhythmias

No method of examination can replace the ECG in the differential diagnosis of the arrhythmias. An extremely slow pulse (sinus bradycardia, sinoatrial block, A V block, idioventricular rhythm) or a rapid pulse (sinus tachycardia, paroxysmal supraventricular tachycardia or atrial flutter, ventricular tachycardia) require an ECG just as initial irregularities of sudden onset (extrasystoles of identical or different origin, atrial fibrillation). Sudden pulselessness during circulatory arrest, Stokes-Adams attack, can be caused either by complete cessation or a very rapid rate of ventricular contraction (e.g., due to ventricular tachycardia). In both types of these rare attacks, the periphery receives an insufficient blood supply. The correct ECG diagnosis may be vital for therapy.

16.2 Diagnosis of Infarction

The objective establishment, localization and observation of the course of an infarction is another important domain of ECG. This must be qualified at once by stating that the ECG diagnosis fails in about 10% of recent and about 50% of old infarcts. The typical changes in depolarization (QRS) and repolarization (ST-T), which are expected of an ECG to establish the diagnosis, sometimes occur only after days. A severe anginal attack suspected to be due to infarction, an acute syndrome (leukocytosis, increased sedimentation rate, fever), and raised transaminase values will be a guide to instituting therapy even before a typical ECG is obtained. Comparative studies on the reliability of enzyme tests and ECG within 24 h of an attack showed that on average the ECG was the more helpful, and particularly in the early stages of infarction, when a high percentage of enzymes may still be negative.

16.3 Suspected Hypertrophy of Individual Parts of The Heart

The ECG may be a valuable adjuvant to radiography, phonocardiogram and other methods in the differential diagnosis of congenital and acquired valvar disease. In mitral stenosis the ECG can present a characteristic combination of signs of left atrial (P mitrale) and right ventricular hypertrophy (vertical axis deviation, typical changes in depolarization and repolarization over the right precordium) which permits a tentative diagnosis from the tracings alone. The ECG of chronic cor pulmonale is also almost specific to the expert. The attempt has been made to distinguish on ECG certain hemodynamically produced forms of hypertrophy (pressure or systolic and volume or diastolic overload). But this has proved possible with some qualification only in the early stages of uncomplicated and typical heart lesions.

What diagnostic support is wrongly expected from the ECG?

What does the ECG not do?

Not fulfilled are all expectations of the ECG in the assessment and differentiation of morphologic and functional changes in the myocardium, its vascularization, and its metabolism. The changes in ST-T are mostly ambiguous. (This is understandable if the "poverty of expression" of repolarization is considered. The ST segment can only be elevated or depressed, and the T wave can vary only between positive and negative.) The causes of all repolarization changes are usually highly complex. In the individual case an extracardial change of myocardial function (e.g., due to a labile autonomic nervous system) cannot always be distinguished from primary cardiac muscle injury due to morphologic changes (e.g., coronary arteriosclerosis), although this may be possible from serial observations. Even electrolyte imbalance (e.g., hypokalemia) rarely provides a specific and typical pattern in the ECG.

The novice falls into the pit more easily than the previously "bitten" expert. In the first instance, artifacts should be mentioned: the most common probably is reversal of electrode connections. This was our own experience of the ECG of a young physician who suffered iatrogenic, cardiac symptoms as a result of such an error. The electrode connections of leads I had been exchanged and the inverted QRS complex in I simulated an anterior wall infarct. The whole tracing was of relatively low voltage with tremor artifacts so that the false recording was not immediately obvious.

Pitfalls of ECG assessment

Another pitfall: inadequate correlation of ECG findings with the clinical picture. For instance, there are harmless extrasystoles of extracardial origin. But electrocardiographically similar extrasystoles may be signs of heart failure in cardiac patients or indicate digitalis toxicity. Among conduction disorders, an incomplete right bundle branch block may be a harmless incidental finding during examination of adolescents for sports activities. But the same bundle branch block has quite another and serious significance if it is encountered in a young person during rheumatic carditis or in an older person due to a septal infarct. On the other hand, surprises occur when the pathologist demonstrates cardiac changes that are in no way reflected in the ECG. This applies particularly to some types of diffuse myocardial fibrosis where a normal ECG obscured the true myocardial situation.

A further important point is neglect of the normal range of the ECG. Those concerned with the ECG and different age will be astonished that conduction times in childhood are shorter by half than in adults. Also axis deviations, definitely diagnosed as pathologic in adults, are normal for infants. The "physiologic right hypertrophy" of young children is well known. Abnormal tracings in advanced age, which frequently reveal slight ST depression and flat T waves, or low voltage, are not always prognostically unfavorable. Extracardial changes can also be the cause of pathologic tracings, as in pulmonary emphysema.

It would be too much to detail all the pitfalls that may be hidden in each ECG deflection. An especially important one seems to be the Q wave whose depth and width causes concern. A Q3 of more than 25% of the R amplitude deep and over 0.04 s wide urgently rouses suspicion of a posterior wall infarct. However, this suspicion must be borne out by a similar pattern in leads aVF, II, and III during deep inspiration. This is the only way to distinguish axis-dependent Q3 waves from those of an infarct, quite apart from the fact that corresponding changes in repolarization are required for infarction to be definite.

At the end of these cautions the banal axiom finds its place again that only the combination of clinical picture, ECG and serial observations permit accurate assessment of ECG findings. It is foolhardy to make a diagnosis from a single ECG or even give a prognosis.

Causes of iatrogenic ECG damage

Several reasons may be adduced for iatrogenic ECG damage, which is still common:

a) Nowadays technologic assistance in medicine is overestimated by laymen and doctors and overvalued against the results of direct examination of patients and eliciting the history. Too much faith is placed in the resting ECG as a method of cardiac diagnosis. The master of American cardiology, P. D. White, has said that a cardiovascular diagnosis is composed of 50% of history, 30% clinical examination, 10% ECG, 5% radiology, and 5% other laboratory aids.

b) The tendency to "have an ECG taken quickly" in order to assuage one's own conscience and that of the attending doctor is promoted — in

148

these times of genuine and supposed lack of time — by the little expenditure of time required for an ECG and foolproof modern equipment. Proper ECG examination, performed by the doctor himself, is not all that short and cannot be done "by the way".

c) A misleading ECG terminology and careless parlance (also in medical reports and ECG findings) are another reason why there are "cardiac patients without cardiac disease." Some terms in the ECG report are bound to be misunderstood by the patient, if he has a chance to see them. For instance, the common expression "myocardial injury" is unfortunate. This expression became accepted in the first few years of ECG to describe changes in repolarization. Originally it meant a general abnormality during repolarization. Such a change may be due to organic disease of the myocardium or a harmless and transient functional alteration in myocardial metabolism. But this expression is accepted by the layman as a final diagnosis of carditis or coronary disease. The same applies to the ECG diagnosis "coronary insufficiency." Also, "physiologic" and "incomplete" right bundle branch block cause much harm if not properly explained to the patient. It is better to speak of an RSR' type in V1, as has been suggested (p. 136).

d) Still another cause of ECG misinterpretation comes from overrating the objectivity of ECG findings and underestimating the subjective factor of any ECG interpretation. The Postgraduate Medical School in London made a valuable contribution to this in 1958:

From one hundred ECG of adult clinical patients, all written with the same photoelectric apparatus and a minimum program of nine leads (standard, Goldberger, V1, V3, V5), 25 normal, 50 cases of infarct, and 25 other abnormal curves were selected. They were randomized twice at a minimum interval of 14 days and submitted for evaluation without clinical data to nine ECG experts and a renowned noncardiologist. Only the terms "normal", "infarct", "abnormal without infarct" were permitted. The result was alarming. The nine experts agreed on only 39 curves, a further 39 curves had a two-thirds majority, and opinions on the remaining 22 ECG diverged (in part considerably). On average, one of eight curves was assessed differently by the same assessors at a second attempt. The results of the nonexpert were entirely out of place. The evidenced uncertainty and personal variability of ECG diagnosis included normal cases, infarct curves, and other anomalies in equal fashion. As far as ascertainable, the reasons for the different opinions were, in the first instance, the pattern of the ventricular complexes in III and aVF, followed by the shape of the initial ventricular deflection in aVL. Authors and editors are united in a warning against irresponsible belittling of difficulties that are inherent in any ECG judgment and advise urgently great caution in diagnostic conclusions based on a single ECG. Very frequently, unequivocal decisions are impossible and in some cases, only a minor diagnostic value can be attached to the curve.

e) Last, but not least, insufficient practice and inclination to dilettantism have to be mentioned as a cause of many ECG misinterpretations.

The many pitfalls of ECG that have been listed can be avoided only by much experience. But can this be achieved? After many years experience with the 1-weekly ECG courses, we continue to believe in following views:

1. Not only the expert physician is in a position correctly to assess an ECG, but every doctor especially interested and trained in cardiology.

But the only doctor who can evaluate an ECG with a clear conscience — and this is *more* than electrophysiologic assessment — is the one who knows the patient or has examined him.

2. In addition to the study of different ECG books specialty education requires:

a) Several systematic ECG refresher courses, tutorials and seminars, preferably with different teachers.

b) Practical training over many months at a medical department with ample opportunities for cardiologic investigations.

It remains to be discussed whether at the end of such a course a test is desirable or not. Participants in our courses have been equally divided in their views.

As a proven method of further self-education we recommend the assessment of tracings in any suitable ECG atlas by covering the explanatory text and then checking oneself, daily or at least at weekends.

Subject-Index

E. K. Chung

Ambulatory Electro-cardiography: Holter Monitor Electrocardiography

1979. Approx. 152 figures, 11 tables. XI, 241 pages
ISBN 3-540-90360-7

Ambulatory (Holter monitor) electrocardiography has been one of the most essential and useful non-invasive diagnostic tools in the field of cardiovascular disease in the pase decade.

The primary indication of ambulatory electrocardiography is cardiac arrhythmia, particularly when the rhythm disturbance occurs transiently or intermittently and transiently, it is impossible to document them on the conventional 12-lead, electrocardiogram (10 second electrical activity recording). Obviously, the advantage of using a 24-hour tape is that any rhythm abnormality which occurs within this time period can be recorded. The purpose of this book is to practical information regarding Holter monitor electrocardiography to assist the physician in improving his diagnostic and therapeutic approach towards cardiac patients. Every known cardiac rhythm problem frequently encountered in daily practice is presented. The book contains 100 actual case studies, each including 12-lead ECG tracing, Holter monitor ECG rhytm strips, and a short case history. In addition, the exercise electrocardiograms (treadmill stress ECG testing) are provided whenever clinically pertinent.

All primary physicians, including family physicians, emergency room physicians, internists, cardioligists, cardiology fellows and medical residents will find this book to be an invaluable aid to their medical practice. Medical students and coronary care unit nurses will also derive benefit from reading this practical and therapeutic guide.

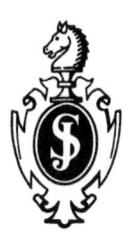

Springer-Verlag
Berlin
Heidelberg
New York

Family Medicine Principles and Practice

Editor: R. B. Taylor

Associate Editors: J. L. Buckingham, E. P. Donatelle, W. E. Jacott, M. G. Rosen

1978. 204 figures, 176 tables. XXXIX, 1365 pages
ISBN 3-540-90303-8

Contents: The Family Physician. Family Medicine Education. Health Care Delivery. – The Patient. The Familiy. Behavior and Counseling. – Principles of Family Medicine: Clinical Evaluation. Clinical Approach to Problems. – Practice of Family Medicine: Planning for Family Practice. Facets of Family Practice. Interactions. Family Practice Today and Tomorrow.

This is one of the most comprehensive textbooks of family medicine ever compiled. It is intended as a reference source of factual data about peoble in health and illness, presented as the approach of the family physician to clinical problems. There is a blend of fact and philosophy, theory and practice, and the book tells not only how to assess the family in crisis, calculate the fluid requirement of a person with serious burns, take a sexual history, and plan the diet for a diabetic, but also how to apply for hospital privileges, plan an office X-ray installation, and guide the patient to available community resources.

Discussed are the diagnosis and management of hundreds of clinical entities encompassing the full spectrum of health care, with guidelines to those problems the family physician should treat indepently, share with a consultant, of refer for definitve care while providing a supportive role to the patient and family. Written for the family doctor, the book contains information useful for the medical student and vital for the practicing general practitioner.

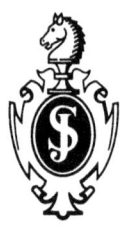

Springer-Verlag
Berlin
Heidelberg
New York